Confessions of a Fat Guy

Scott Moss

Published by Scott Moss, 2024.

While every precaution has been taken in the preparation of this book, the publisher assumes no responsibility for errors or omissions, or for damages resulting from the use of the information contained herein.

CONFESSIONS OF A FAT GUY

First edition. November 8, 2024.

Copyright © 2024 Scott Moss.

ISBN: 979-8227545497

Written by Scott Moss.

Table of Contents

Confessions of a Fat Guy 1

Chapter 31 | This section is for older teens and adults. If you are younger than this I ask that you please wait to read this until you're at least 16. You'll understand what this chapter means when you're older. So please move on to the next chapter so you can get the full value of this book. Please do this for me. 108

To everyone who knows the ups and downs of weight loss.

Confessions of a Fat Guy
By Scott W. Moss
Dedication. Please take the time to read this before you buy this book.

I'd like to dedicate this book to all the children, adolescents, young teenagers, older teenagers, and adults who have struggled with weight problems. Most of you may have had a weight problem for some time now. Maybe since you were a little kid. This is the make-or-break time for you. I'm not one of those screaming exercise freaks or a nasty diet person who says, "If you only eat celery for the rest of your life, you'll lose weight." I can't stand those kinds of people. I will put in very simple terms what you need to do to lose weight and feel fantastic after-effects when the weight is gone. This is my story. It's not always happy, but I do have kind of a warped sense of humor so it should be a fun read. In case someone hasn't said this in a while to you, I love you. It doesn't matter if you're overweight. I know what you have inside of you. I hope I can make your life easier by starting you off on a weight loss and life journey so you can live long enough to be a burden to your kids.

Prologue

I've had both a wonderful and difficult life. I found a new term that explains the difficult times I've had to endure because I've been overweight. The newest term used is being fat-shamed. I've been fat-shamed for all but about 10 years of my life. I'm 61 years old. I have been married to a wonderful woman for 38 years. She is one of those special people who said she would love me through the good times and the bad times. If me being significantly overweight would be considered the "bad times" then she is a saint. Right up there with the lovely Mother Theresa. Ok, maybe that's a stretch. Mother Theresa was never married to a fat guy. Eileen has been. That's a step above most of the saints.

It has to be difficult to be married to someone who is morbidly obese now who wasn't when we got married. I was 210 pounds when we got married. I'm 6'2" in height so I'm naturally a big guy. I was a hockey player. Did a lot of weightlifting way back then too. I wasn't huge, but I was well-defined. I will eventually get into the way I became thin after being 290 pounds in high school. I had been fat-shamed since I was in 5th grade. You can imagine all the nicknames I acquired over the years. I will try to recall them throughout this book, but I am sure I will forget some. The most popular one was Fat Moss. Let's just forgo my first name and replace it with fat. Talk about fat shaming. The others will be listed in the upcoming chapters. I'm sure you'll be familiar with most of them. Hopefully, you will not have been called these names as much as I was.

This book is for both women and men. It is an autobiography, not a how-to book. I hope it will inspire you, sure. But more than anything, I want you to see how a life unfolds while spending most of a life overweight.

Chapter 1

Before the fat explosion

I should let you know right away that I am 61 years old. Why does this matter? Because I've had a lifetime of experience. I know what it's like to be in great physical shape, and I also know what it's like to be 150 pounds overweight. I can tell you from experience what you'll go through if you remain overweight. I hate the word fat. Especially when it's used to describe a person. It's heartless. The newest term that I find to be extremely accurate when it comes to how people treat someone who is overweight is called being fat-shamed. If I went around saying "Hey pizza face" to someone with a bad acne problem my parents would have kicked my ass. But yet my own grandmother once said, "what did that fat ass do this time?" She used it to describe a fall down I had down the stairs that caused a fractured elbow. My own grandmother! What a piece of work. She was the absolute grand champion of guilt. She was nasty, vindictive, and just plain mean to her own family. She also by pure osmosis trained my mother extremely well, putting her in a close second. This is the kind of person that was the pot calling the kettle black. She had to be 50 pounds overweight. I guess you get a pass when you're old. Nobody had the guts to fat-shame her. I know my dad was never happy with the way she treated my mother. But she was one of the people who fat-shamed me. And her endeavor in it was brutal. Not to mention she was my fricken grandma!

I started out thin. A normal kid with normal height and weight ratios. I started school as a normal kid. My grades were good. Although later on, I did find out I had a mild learning disability where I ignored the first letter of a word. Putting things in alphabetical order was hard for me. It only appears now when I type too fast. I just forget to put the first letter of the word. Other than that, things were good.

I played outside in all four seasons. I live just southwest of Chicago. So, football and hockey were as popular as baseball and basketball. I also had a great time sledding, always looking for a bigger hill. My dad could find them like a bloodhound. They always ended up in the trees, though. I wonder sometimes if he was trying to cut the food bill down by getting rid of one of us. No one played soccer back then. Remember, I'm 61. I have nothing against soccer. In fact, soccer players have to be in much better shape than most players in any other sport. But back when I was a kid, soccer hadn't hit the United States as it has now. These sports were a big part of my life, and it would remain that way until the pain began its slow assault on me. Some of that pain was due to the sport itself. But I think a lot of it was because of the extra weight I carried while playing that sport that caused a good deal of damage.

Let's quickly talk about what kind of damage the body endures when you are overweight during the decades of life. Let's start with your childhood.

During childhood, most of the problems are because of your peers causing you distress because of the name-calling that goes along with being heavy. Kids are cruel. They fold under peer pressure very easily. One bully will start calling you names and the rest of the kids in class will follow his or her lead. It usually starts with one of the pretty people. The guy every girl likes, or the girl every guy likes. I don't know why this happens, it's not like we were a threat to their looks. No one was looking at me when I got heavy. So why the name-calling? Just because they could. I wonder sometimes if this was a learned activity. Did these kids grow up in environments that were laden with prejudice? Maybe they had the perfect parents. You know the ones. Mom was a beauty queen and dad was the captain of the football team. They looked perfect and thought everyone else was below them, so it was ok to teach their child to do the same thing they did. When confronted by another parent about name-calling, they couldn't believe their little Johnny could be so mean. It was impossible. Clueless people. Your little Johnny was an ass. He probably still is. And both of his parents are now fat, and they get shit about it all the time and it makes me happy.

Chapter 2

The beginning of the end

When I got to 4th grade things were still good. I was 10 years old because I had an early birthday. The cutoff was December 2nd, and I was born on the fourth, so I started school so that I was the oldest kid in class. It was the first year I had a male teacher. He was right out of the late 60s with long curly hair and a full beard. If you're young you probably won't remember the band Styx. They sang Renegade and Blue-Collar Man. They play those songs a lot at hockey and football games. The steelers football team has a third-quarter tribute with the song "Renegade" in it. Anyway, my teacher looked exactly like the lead singer of Styx in the early years of the band. His name was different, and I know he never changed it. It was a popular look back then, and it fit him. He did have a temper. Also liked to put his feet up on the desk when he taught. That's about all I remember. He was a pretty cool guy, though. He would always pick me as one of the captains in whatever sport we were playing in gym class. I didn't get a full-time gym teacher till 5th grade. More about him later. He ended up playing a big part in my life, so I don't want to leave him out. 4th grade was the last grade for me to be in the cool kid group. All because I was thin like the other boys in the group.

Now, here's where things get ugly. And by ugly, I mean me. Things had changed at my household drastically between 4th and 5th grade. That summer was one of the great changes in my household. I should start with a little backstory. My dad was a salesman. Mainly nuts, bolts, fasteners, and washers. Industrial stuff. Back then $20,000 wasn't a bad salary for a salesman. He had the personality to be a good one but every time he would start to make more money in a job with sales bonuses or just increasing the customer base, they would fire him because he was making too much money. He would get kicked back down to $20,000 again and have to start over until the same thing happened. He wanted to start his own business, but my mom had very little to no faith in that. She made it clear to him that it was not an option. She needed him to have a steady paycheck. I think it was a big mistake. Actually, a monumental mistake. My mom and dad had 5 kids. Why does that matter? Because he could have had a team of cheap slave labor just from his kids. I believe he had the ambition to do it and the need. Raising 5 kids is not cheap. Even way back then. Starting his own business would have been a way out of the lower middle class we were in. I had faith in my father even way back then. He always went to work and came home later than he was required to be at work. He drove all over the Chicagoland area checking in on accounts, getting new orders, and always working hard for the owner of the business he was working for. After he would set up all these new accounts, they would fire him and put someone in his position just to maintain the new accounts he added to the business. I wish I could remember some of his boss's names, I'd out them and risk the lawsuits.

I owned my own business for 20+ years. Some months you don't make a lot of money. It's just the nature of the beast. Some weeks I made $6000 and the next week I might make $600. I think my dad went through the same thing in sales. But to put a second mortgage on the house to start his own business was out of the question because of my mother. He was so deeply in love with my mother that he wouldn't do anything to make her be disappointed with him. Although because of my mother's black belt in guilt, they fought like hell. My dad walked around the house with a very confused look on his face for most of my childhood and teenage years. He never knew what he did wrong. Sometimes I think his anger toward her was transferred to his quick hand across our asses. Spanking was common back then too. Be glad you live now where they know that it is not a good idea to beat a child.

Sorry, off on a tangent. Back to our regularly scheduled programming. My mom got a full-time job at the Lions Club of America. That full-time job also included travel. She went to Taiwan once. And many other places I can't remember. With her new job, a problem occurred. They had 5 kids and now both of them were working. My mom had stayed home with us since we were born. Well, what happens when both parents work, and you can't afford a babysitter that will be there all week from 9 to 5? That's right children! Put the oldest child in that role whether he likes it or not. Who was that oldest child? That's right! It was me. I was 10 years old. My mom started the job at the beginning of summer between 4th and 5th grade. I was in charge of a 9-year-old, an 8-year-old, a 5-year-old, and a very angry 3-year-old. She wanted her mommy. Not a very poor substitute. So, imagine, you're 10 years old and have to stay home every day watching all these kids. The most I could do was take the 5 and 3-year-olds down to the park and watch them play. I couldn't even get on a swing because the 5-year-old was climbing the 15-foot monkey bars while the 3-year-old was putting rocks in her mouth. My two other siblings were able to go out, ride their bikes, and play with their friends. I made them come home for lunch just to make sure they were still alive. Usually, my dad would come home first at about 5:00. My mom at 5:30. I couldn't go anywhere until we ate dinner and did the dishes.

That put it at about 6:30. I could go out after that for about an hour and a half. I had to be in bed by 9:00. That gave me about an hour to get home because I would have to shower at night and then go to bed. 1 hour of free time for a 10-year-old is not nearly enough. I was angry. Real angry. My parents had completely dropped this bomb on me taking away any chance of a normal summer with my friends.

So, what do you do when you're chained to 5 kids at the age of 10? You get incredibly bored and start to eat anything in sight. Still, all on me for eating that much but you know what boredom does to kids. They usually get in trouble. That's what I was doing. Eating enough food to piss them off. Their grocery bill went up significantly. I always went grocery shopping with my mom so I could guilt trip her into everything I wanted to eat that week. I was already a yellow belt in guilt so I could sell it pretty well.

My dad started bringing home two gallons of milk every night. You see, I hate pop or soda depending on where you're from. It never tasted good to me. I liked cherry Kool-Aid but that had tons of sugar in it too. I loved milk. I loved chocolate milk so bad I asked it to marry me. Labels on food and milk or pop were not required back then. And even if you told me that a portion of food was high in carbohydrates, I would have no idea what you meant. Here's a little fact I pulled about food labels: *Nutrition information was not always required on packaged foods and beverages prior to 1990. The U.S. Nutrition Facts label first appeared in 1994 and was revised in 2016. A newer, more updated version is required on products as of January 1, 2020.* I found this at the website foodinsight.org. There is a lot of great information on that site so check it out when you get the chance.

Chapter 3

The tragedy continues

Back then milk delivery services still available. It was too expensive for my parents, so we didn't have it. But my parents were giving me a whopping 10 dollars a week to watch 4 kids. When I saw the dixie milk truck coming down our street because I knew what day and time he was going to be there down to the minute, I would wave him down and buy a quart of chocolate milk. It was all of 50 cents so with the money I made I could buy about 2 to 3 quarts a week. To make it last longer I would mix the chocolate milk with the remaining white milk and that was designated as my gallon from that point on. And one other thing. There wasn't 1 or 2 percent milk. It was vitamin D 4% milk fat. You could hit me with a car even today and none of my bones would break. I'm not going to try that out for you.

During my trips to the grocery store, I would land in one aisle that my mom would have to go slowly through. Let's just put it this way. Little Debbie and I had quite a relationship. We went out together for many years. She made me so happy I asked her to marry me. With her Starcrunch, Swiss Rolls, Zebra Cakes, Chocolate Cupcakes, Powdered Mini Donuts, Frosted Mini Donuts, Nuddy Buddy Wafer Bars, Peanut Butter Crunch Bars blah blah blah. If they made it, I ate it. I also had to make a stop at the candy aisle because when you're an overweight child, it's the law.

Next came the cereal aisle. I was allowed three boxes a week which I was supposed to share with my brothers and sisters. In a dictatorship, which was the way I ran the house, the head honcho gets the lion's share of the cereal. My mom bought at least 5 boxes of cereal a week. Some of my favorites were anything with sugar in it. Frosted Flakes, Capt. Crunch, Cocoa Pebbles, Cocoa Puffs, Count Chocula (A personal favorite), Lucky Charms, Cookie Crisps, Honey Nut Cheerios with extra sugar on top, Golden Crisps, which was originally called Sugar Crisps. Fruit Loops were the closest thing I ever got to actual fruit. Putting away the groceries when we got home could take as long as going through the grocery store did. Extra cereal went on top of the fridge where I was the only one that could reach it. Do know how high in carbohydrates cereal is? So that didn't help at all either.

So, between eating all this food and drinking all that milk in about 5 months I put on 50 pounds. As a fricken 10-year-old! When it was time to go back to school my parents had my neighbor watch my little sister and the rest of us went to the same school. We could and did walk to school, no matter what it was doing outside. I remember thinking my friends are going to have a field day with me. And I was right. I hadn't seen them all summer, so they were in shock when they saw me. The names started not too long after that. I remember standing in line waiting for my fifth-grade class to go into school when the kid behind me said "I can't even see the teacher because this fat ass is right in front of me!" So, on day one, I had to defend myself from these fat hating people. One of the things I noticed when I got heavy was that my strength increased. Carrying around 50 extra pounds day after day will make you strong. I pushed let's call him "Fred" so hard that he hit the ground hard enough to need 3 stitches in the back of his head. I noticed pretty quickly after that incident was I knew I had an anger problem. The first day of school and I'm in trouble. I told them that someone pushed me, and I bumped into Fred. The principal bought it, so I didn't have to serve any time. Fred never said anything bad to me for the next 2 years. Then he went to a different junior high. So, if you're reading this Fred, I'm really sorry for hurting you but I did teach you a lesson about being nice to everyone.

The name-calling was brutal. I heard it from everyone, including my best friends. Guys I had played baseball with last summer were calling me names and grabbing my stomach to shake it. When I gained weight, my legs stayed normal, but my torso got chubby. Forgot about that word. Heard that one from some of my previous teachers. Let's see if I can remember some of the names I got called. I started with fat ass and chubby so let's go from there. Big ass, fatty, and of course the song that went with it. Let's everybody sing it! Fatty, fatty two-by-four, can't get through the bathroom door, so he makes it on the floor. Fatty fatty two by four. Oh, the memories. That one always occurred in front of the girls in my class for some reason. Let's continue with the names. Lard ass, lumpy, tubby, porker, fatso, elephant, chubster, chunky monkey, fattie, lardo, land whale, oinker, fat pig, pudge (used rather effectively by my uncles), thunder thighs, man boobs, look at those love handles, and my personal favorite big fat slob. Pretty painful to listen to, isn't it? Especially if you were one of those name callers and now, your fat, and people call you these names. Karma is a bitch. But I'm happy that it hit you as hard as it hit me as a kid. Being a kid when all these names are not only hurtful, they make you into one of two things. A crier or a fighter. I became a fighter. A nasty as-hell fighter. And no, I didn't sit on any of my opponents. I wanted to hurt some of my good friends, but I also didn't want to lose them either. I tolerated their jokes for a short period of time. If they finally crossed the line, I could just give them a look and they'd stop. These were close friends in 4th grade. Now they had a different agenda. It was making fun of Scott season and I was the elephant they were hunting. So, to Rick, Leon, Rich, Tony, Jimbo, Kim, Cheryl, Kathy, Sandy, and many others I don't remember this book is also dedicated to you. I hope you're all fat now and have to buy your clothes at the big and tall shop or at Lane Bryant. It's only fair.

Chapter 5
Still can play sports

The one thing I wouldn't let suffer because of my weight was my abilities in sports. I couldn't run as fast anymore, so if we were playing baseball and I should have had a double I had to settle for a single. But now, with all the extra body weight I added I also had a lot of muscle from carrying it around. I could hit the hell out of a baseball. My slapshot in hockey sent people dancing out of the way sometimes including the goalie, and as for football, I could run anyone down. I couldn't run for long, but it usually took about three guys to bring me down. I could block just about anyone. As for basketball, I had to work on my outside shot because I didn't have the speed to charge in without fouling someone. In high school, I got charged with an offensive foul at least 3 times a game. But I still tried. My outside shot was good, so I used that as a weapon. Now pole vaulting was out of the question as was the 100-yard sprint. Let's just say anything involving track. I even had trouble with the shotput. I knew where it was going but I couldn't get the stepping and body movements right. As for the discus, I caused fear and destruction with that almost immediately. I remember putting a huge dent in one of the aluminum sheds that housed the outsid track equipment.

But the thing is I tried to do everything I did before. I wasn't going to sit there and feel sorry for myself. I was going to show everyone that I was still a decent athlete. Especially in hockey because that was my sport. The one I liked the best. I never stopped skating. I wasn't lightning fast, and I would tire fast but when I was out there, they got all of me.

In 5th grade, we got a gym teacher. The grade school I went to didn't have a gym teacher until then. He was a little bit of a hard ass but most of them are. He didn't give me a hard time about being fat but he did help me get more active by showing me some exercises I could do and said I should just try to go for a long walk once a day. This guy's name is Bill LeMonnier[1]. If it sounds familiar, you may know him as one of the best referees in college football. I'm talking about national championship games. He has turned down refereeing in the NFL because he doesn't want to deal with a bunch of overpaid millionaires that think they can give him shit.

Mr. LeMonnier taught us about physical fitness. He didn't make fun of the kids that weren't physically fit. He would encourage us. Even going as far as telling me to try to eat more fruits and vegetables if I wanted to be a pro hockey player. That was my dream back then. It remained my dream until a very large defenseman fell across my knee when I was playing goalie and blew it out. Dream over. At that time, I was practicing with a college team three nights a week. Who was my

---

1. https://www.youtube.com/watch?v=XxsVUkAVvkU

coach? Bill LeMonnier. He would even come and pick me up to take me to practice during my senior year of high school. With his help, I got offered some scholarships to some pretty nice colleges. Not that I could afford to go, mind you. They weren't full-ride scholarships, and my parents just didn't have the money. He was a big part of my life at that time. Then one day after I had 4 kids, and they were old enough for me to sit down and watch a college football game, they do a close-up shot of the referee during a call on the field. I hear the voice, turn around and who is it? Bill LeMonnier. He had a long and illustrious career in college football and I'm glad I can say I know him.

Off on a tangent there but it's important for 6th grade. Because he found out that I could shoot a hockey puck like nobody's business. We were goofing around in gym class with some lightweight hockey equipment. Plastic blades with a lightweight puck. He put little strips of wood down the shafts of the sticks so they wouldn't bend. It was floor hockey at its finest. And he wanted to start an after-school league. He called out during gym class that the league would start soon. He picked two captains. One was my close friend Leon and the other one was someone I don't remember. I thought Leon would pick me first or second to be on his team. As the picks went on, Leon didn't seem to want to pick me. I was second to last to be picked. And it wasn't by Leon. The other guy picked me. I was really hurt. All my so-called "friends" were on Leon's team. I was the only one on the other guy's team and I was pissed. I was going to show them all that they made a mistake. Sometimes anger can be the best motivator.

The league was set up, so we played once a week until winter break. My captain quit 2 games in, so they made me the captain. There were about 6 teams in the league. Mr. LeMonnier kept a couple of charts on the walls of the gym to see where each team stood. The other list showed the top goal scorer. We had 5 games in total. I lead the top scorer all 5 weeks. I wanted to get back at my friends. When we played them, I worked even harder to win, just to get revenge. We were tied with Leon's team for the final game. I vaguely remember scoring 11 goals in 30 minutes. I'd like to say we won but that would be a lie. We lost by one goal. But I was still proud of my team's work. None of them wanted to be hockey players. They were there for the fun of it. I did win the award for the most goals scored. I averaged over 10 goals a game. No one was even near me in that department. Leon told me after the final game that he was sorry he didn't pick me. He thought I wouldn't be fast enough. Big mistake. But I forgave him. But it was another example of prejudice against overweight people. I'd like to say that was the last time that happened, but I would go through that so many more times.

Chapter 6

Junior high school

Nothing like walking into a new school with an extra 50 pounds on me. This school was diversified. About 50/50. All the parents were afraid of us going there because there were black kids at the junior high. The generation before mine was so prejudiced it was incredible. I never felt out of place at junior high. I had black and white friends. It never mattered to me. The only thing I did notice was the black kids didn't make fun of me for being fat. The white kids did. Including some of the white teachers. The school was so much bigger than our grade school. It was a so the first time we moved from classroom to classroom. I loved being in a class with different people every hour. The problem with that though was there was a new group of kids every hour to make fun of me. That's when I became the kid you didn't mess with. Someone called me fat ass in the hallway, and I grabbed him by the shirt and slammed him into a locker. The hallway was filled with kids including 8th graders. I was bigger than most of them too. I just needed to make one person an example. Go ahead and make fun of me. I can do this to you if you want to call me names. As you can see, anger was an issue too. Some overweight people take the shit, others didn't. I definitely fell into the didn't category. It was bad enough taking the disgusted looks from the girls. I would never touch a girl that made fun of me. I might have a quick comment back at her to completely embarrass her in front of everyone.

I was also developing a quick wit and a sense of humor. When you are overweight, you have to develop something that will make it easier to fit in. My dad had a great sense of humor, so it wasn't hard for me to pick up on this. Making people laugh was the best way to get them on my side. Most of the time it worked. But when you're that age in a new school you just tried to get through the day. They kept the eighth graders away from the seventh graders so it was rare that I would have to deal with them.

I did make a friend for life in junior high. I met a guy named Jeff and we hit it off right away. He just happened to be one of the best-looking guys in the school. I was hoping for some of his cast off's but that didn't happen. Jeff played on the basketball team, was in a band (if you want to call it that) and he could talk his way into any girl's heart by just smiling at her. I was just a satellite rotating around him. Jeff was the moon to all the girls in junior high. He would get asked out all the time. Mind you going out meant your mom or dad dropping you off at the mall and maybe holding hands.

So, I guess I wasn't missing much. But hanging around with him gave me lessons on how to be cool with girls. Unfortunately, no girls were standing in line for me. I was regularly told I was too fat. I could barely fit into the chair with the attached desktop. I could wear my uncle's air force uniform top over a shirt. Meaning, I couldn't button it. He wasn't very big, but he was still an adult. I was 13 years old. I don't know how much I weighed, but I had to be pushing 200 pounds. By eighth grade, I must have weighed 220. I was still making everyone laugh and Jeff and I had a good time whatever we did. Other than the name-calling and complete rejections, things were good.

I was lucky enough to have two great teachers in those years. One was a cool social studies teacher. The other was a very strict history teacher. He was extremely tough to have as a teacher, but I have to thank him for my love of history. And the social studies teacher taught me about life. They both came to my wedding many years later. That's how close I was to them. I got to watch Jeff's band get better and better. When their lead singer couldn't make it to practice, I would fill in for him. I was a good singer and if I had the look that a lead singer needs, I may have been considered for the job of the lead singer. I had more of a bodyguard body. There have only been a handful of prominent big lead singers in rock and roll. The one I looked like more than any of them was Meatloaf (born Marvin Lee Aday; September 27, 1947 – January 20, 2022). His voice and talent on stage were absolutely fantastic. But unfortunately, I wasn't going to be given the chance to be one of those big lead singers.

Chapter 7

High school

Ahhhh! The beauty of high school is when you're an overweight guy who now had developed a mild to moderate acne problem. And how prey tell do you think it is for said student? Nothing but relentless teasing and rejection.

My high school was in Tinley Park, IL. At the time, Tinley Park was so white that the ground could sense when a black man was near and would call the cops. (yes, It was that prejudice) Not the most opened minded folks in the late 70s or early 80s. I was bussed to Tinley from my hometown of Oak Forest, IL, and my town wasn't any better. When I started there my freshman year there were just a handful of black kids and even fewer Hispanic kids in my high school. Most of them had gone to my junior high school so I knew them. They had to endure threats, fights, and bigotry like you wouldn't believe. I watched a black kid get stabbed and a white girl throw a punch at a black girl. She missed and shattered the glass next to a classroom door. They had to rush her to the hospital because she had cut up her hand and wrist so badly. The white girl started the fight with a racial slur and ended up in an ambulance—poetic justice at its finest. The black kids were just trying to survive in a white high school. By senior year, most of them were just regular friends like the white kids. I still knew prejudiced white kids, but they were finally starting to be a dying breed by senior year.

Let's go back to freshman year. I decided (actually, my best friend decided) that I wanted to play football. During freshman year no one was cut from the team. If you tried out, you made the team. Unless you were me. We had the most obnoxious coach I had ever had the displeasure of working with. Not that it was working. It was me running laps and him screaming at me because I was fat. He called me every name in the book related to someone being fat. He spared no insult while I was at practice. I have to say I think my favorite at that time was "Lard Ass." This guy was a pain in my ass for most of high school. Did you ever feel that someone had it in for you from day one? For some reason, this was that guy. The guy also kept up his relentless insults and pressure even when I tried out for baseball. He coached my summer baseball team and rarely let me play. During practice, he would whip rubber balls at me to see if I could hit them. Now, mind you this is a full-grown adult throwing a full-sized rubber ball that we could practice with indoors if it was raining or the field was wet. One of the assistant coaches was commenting on my ability to hit the ball hard. Then instead of complimenting me on it, he went out to where the pitcher was and started throwing the ball as hard as he could to see if I could hit off him. Because every freshman should have been able to hit the 26-year-old coaches fast pitching. When he finally hit me with the ball, I picked it up and threw it back at him as quickly as I could. I almost got him in the nuts. I tossed the bat behind me and walked back to the other players. I got a lot of pats on the back. He never said anything to me again. Unfortunately, it cost me playing time. I think if my mother wasn't there bitching one day, he would have never put me in. When he finally did, I had 1 error, 2 base hits, and a home run over the left field fence. But it didn't matter. I was fat and this guy didn't like fat kids. Plain and simple. How do I know? He opened a bar 3 or 4 years after we graduated, and I went there with a bunch of my friends. I was thin and built by then and he didn't recognize me. He stuck out his hand and introduced himself. I said "I know exactly who you are. You're the guy who hated fat kids in high school." of course he denied it. I said "you gave me shit for 4 years. I'm here because my friends wanted to come. Not to see you. And if you can't figure out who I am that makes me think even less of you." He was starting to get a little hot which is what I was going for. He said, "well then who the fuck are you?" I said my name and he just about freaked. He said "shit. I guess you're right. I was always on your ass about your weight. I didn't know what I was doing, and I thought I could motivate you if I gave you shit all the time." I said, "how'd that work out for you?" he said, "Well, by the way, you're looking at me now I'd say it didn't work so well. You look like you're going to jump over the bar and kick my ass. Let me get you a drink on the house and we'll start over." he went to get me a beer and spent the next 15 minutes (the bar wasn't busy and closed down within a year.) trying to apologize for how he treated me. He did have one thing on me. When I tried out for football, he would make me run an extra mile because he was pissed that the first mile I ran took me so long. One day I was having trouble with my knee and had fallen way behind. When I finally got in, he made a show out of yelling at me and calling me a "fat fuck" and that I'd never play for him because I was so fat. I knew he was lying because the assistant coach had already moved me from the offensive line to the defensive end because I was so fast off the snap. The quarterback was a good friend of mine, and we would make a game out of how many times I could sack him vs how many times he could get out of my grasp. We were about 50/50 by the time I quit. How I quit is the best part of this story.

  It was about 95 degrees and 100% humidity. It was also 8:00 in the morning. So, the sun was already blazing. Even the guys that were in shape were dragging on the mile we had to run at the beginning of practice. So, I was basically dying. The group was already doing calisthenics when I finally got in. The head coach got right into my face and started berating me. He was spitting on me every time he yelled. I was getting so incredibly mad that I was about to punch him. The assistant coach pulled him off of me. I turned to him and yelled, "You're the biggest asshole I've ever had the absolute displeasure of meeting." That got a laugh out of all my teammates. I started to walk away. When I was about 10 feet away, he was still giving me shit. I took my helmet off and whipped it at him. It hit him in the shoulder which was a shame because I was going for his face. I kept walking hoping he would come after me because I was going to kill this bastard. The fat slurs were still coming as I did a slow strip tease on the way back to the locker room. I took off my shoulder pads and threw them about 20 yards to the right of me, my jersey went far, and I even took my football pants off and whipped them to the left. I walked into the locker room in my gym shorts. I went to my locker to get dressed when the assistant coach came up to me and begged me not to quit. He said I could play defensive end well and they needed me on the team. I said "I'll play when you become the head coach. So, report this little incident to the athletic director and see if they give you the job and kick that asshole off the field." He tried hard to talk me back onto the field. Even after the team lost its first couple of games. I wasn't having any of it. I did file a complaint against him with the athletic director putting down some of the names he called me along with the extra work he made me do. Well, the athletic director didn't like fat kids either because he never approached me afterward to tell me what happened with the complaint. I'm sure it got placed into the round file cabinet next to his desk. If this coach had treated a kid that way in today's environment, he would have been thrown out on his ear. My teammates would congratulate me in the hallway about how I stood up to him but at the same time be mad that I had quit. I understood why they were mad; I think I would have made that team better. But I could only take so much. All this bullshit is because a coach couldn't or wouldn't deal with an overweight kid on his team. If he had come to me and given me a special diet and spent extra time with me in the weight room, he would have been a decent guy trying to help me get in shape for football. But instead, he just wanted to humiliate me in front of everyone for being fat. I use this word I hate during this section because that's the word he chose to tease me with. Mr. D, I hope you're 50 pounds overweight and have to shop at the big and tall shop. I'd like to see you so I could call you a fat bastard like you did to me. God that felt good to write out.

Chapter 8

Dealing with the upperclassmen and women

When I started school, most of the upperclassmen thought I was older because of my size. Also some of my fighting on the football field had gotten around. I was over 6 feet tall by then and probably weighed 250 pounds. A lot of them thought I had transferred in from another school. That didn't stop the name calling though. It came from all sides. I started to get into some fights because of the name-calling. Mostly me pushing someone into a wall or a locker and then they would come at me, and I would hit them once in the face because I was pretty fast with my fists. They'd fall to the ground, and I'd walk away. That next period I'd be called down to the dean's office and have to tell my side of the story. They would say "just because he called you a name doesn't give you the right to beat him up." You know, covering for the skinny asshole who started the whole thing. I'd get a detention or two and just do my homework during it. When my parents would ask why they had to pick me up I'd make up some lie about helping the art teacher (who was about 22 and absolutely gorgeous) and they'd buy it. Sometimes I would help her after school because I could draw and paint and liked to finish my projects after school sometimes. She was so nice and would work with me and not treat me any differently than any other kid. She even taught me some other forms of art like sculpture and enamel work. I never felt like the fat guy. I felt like a real person in her class. Someone who was respected for my talents. She even let me bring in a cassette tape (yes I'm that old) to play during class. She usually only played her own cassettes. My favorite band was Styx and they had just come out with the Grand Illusion album. It was my absolute favorite. She let us listen to the whole album. She was fantastic. She only stayed during my freshman year. Otherwise, I'm sure we'd have married and had 10 children and 25 grandchildren by now. Back then I would be considered the luckiest man/boy even if she wanted me. Nowadays, she'd be charged with a very bad crime. She never made fun of me and was always so nice. It's a shame she left. I would have liked to work with her for all four years.

The worst name-calling occurred in front of the class. There was one guy named Dave M. Dave never missed the possibility to embarrass me in front of a classroom full of students. He was a little fireplug. Built from weightlifting, being a football player, and being an overall asshole to most people. He saw me as an easy target.

After enduring many a taught in school from this guy in the hallway or in a classroom I finally had enough. We were in my favorite class which was business law with one of the best teachers in the entire high school. I didn't do very well on a question the teacher had asked me when Dave decided to interject and call me a stupid fat ass. I intern called him a muscle head with no brains. He then called me something else and I replied. When he opened his mouth to say one more thing I got up and tossed my chair back to the ground pretty hard. I started to storm up my aisle to get to him across the room. Our teacher Mr. L got in the way and stopped me but just barely. I didn't push Mr. L but I made him stop me with his body. Mr. L was an average-sized guy and had trouble stopping me. By this time Dave was still sitting in his chair with a pretty scared look on his face. If you poke the bear one too many times, he's going to wake up. I woke up. I was second to the last person in the first row of chairs, he was first in the row farthest away from me.

I was going to nail him right out in the hallway after class. That was my plan. What're a couple more detentions? It had been a while since I had to stand up for myself like this. So, what the hell? As the bell went off Mr. L got up and quickly got in front of me, holding me in place until Dave was long gone. He did that for a week. Dave would bolt out of class every time and I had no idea where he was going. He hadn't said anything bad to me all week so after Mr. L blocked me on Friday, he told me the reason he blocked me all week was that "teachers talk. You have a reputation for destroying your opponents. He's built big but you are at least 5 inches taller than him and have about 70 pounds on him. You're going to get blood all over my classroom." He was right. That was exactly what I planned to do. I told Mr. L that if he said something to me in class again, I was going to go right through him to get to Dave. So, give him that message and I'll stop. I saw Mr. L by Dave's desk on Monday of the next week. He was talking to Dave and pointing his finger toward me. I don't know what he said to him, but he never called me another name out loud in class. I caught up to him at a party our senior year and he hadn't grown much. He was still playing football so I knew he would be strong. I walked up to him in the backyard and said "If you say sorry for all the name-calling you did to me junior year, I won't hurt you tonight. He was hammered and I wasn't. He said "I was just fucking with you, Moss. I just wanted to get a rise out of you. I wouldn't have fought you; you would have destroyed me. I was just trying to show off for this girl that was in the class." I said "Who was the girl? He said "Melissa D." Now I knew what Melissa D. looked like and if this was the only way Dave thought he could impress her I guess I understood why he was being such an ass. Pick a fight with the biggest guy in school and if you win it will impress her. I said to Dave "you know I was about to hurt you, didn't you?" He said at the time he was willing to take that chance to impress her. I just shook my head at him. "Why didn't you fight me after class or after school if you were so bent on showing off to her? Dave said "Hell, I didn't want to fight you. I just wanted to look tough in front of her. I knew what would happen if we fought. I might have gotten a few shots in, but I saw you freshman year at football. You threw guys around like they were rag dolls. I'm sorry I was such an ass. She ended up having a boyfriend at another school so none of it would have mattered." I still felt like punching him, but he was so drunk he'd have been out with one punch, and what's the fun in that? He never said anything else to me that whole year. We never had a class together senior year. I hadn't even seen him up until the party. I have a significant problem letting things go. It's still that way today. As you can tell I remember this shit way too long for my own good. But I also can recall good things too. Like some "not-so-good" girls after I did lose the weight. So, it's a double-edged sword. Sometimes it's nice to have a memory like this. I'm trying to bring to the forefront some of the things overweight kids go through in school and as you'll see, some of the things a full-grown adult goes through.

Chapter 9

Parties

Yes, we had parties back then children. Big two-keg parties with Old Style beer. I often wondered how many total cases of toilet paper people went through the next day. I don't think I could drink an Old Style if my life depended on it right now. It started my freshman year. When I was still involved in my very short career as a football player, there was a guy named Rich who had some very old parents. The dad would go buy the keg for the party and as long as we stayed in the garage, his parents were ok with the whole "let's get the 14 and 15-year-olds drunk." We did have fun, but these were for football players only. I thought Rich was a pretty good friend. We hung out during grade school and junior high. The week I threw my helmet at the coach there was a big party at Rich's house planned. When I showed up to go in, my so-called friend Rich said I couldn't go to the parties anymore because I quit football. I asked him if he understood why I quit football. He said he wasn't at practice that day. He said I couldn't come in because I wasn't on the team anymore. I walked away from that house feeling pretty bad. When a good friend betrays you the first thing you think of is "he must not like me because I'm fat." I walked home that night and decided I would find a new bunch of friends. Years later at a party, Rich B. said something nasty to my friend Bill D. Bill came after him and we were able to stop him before he killed Rich. I got the absolute pleasure of throwing Rich out of that party. The last thing I said was "payback can be a bitch. Remember freshman year when you wouldn't let me go to your party because I wasn't playing football anymore? Well, call this karma. Now go home."

I did find the high school comedians and we all bonded. A good portion of them were on the swim team so I'd go watch them to cheer them on which when you think of it, their ears are almost always submerged so they couldn't hear us anyway. I also found a lifelong friend named Bill D. At the writing of this book, I just sent him a movie clip of my grandson trying on a cowboy hat at the age of 18 months. He's such a ham it was hilarious. Bill got a real kick out of it.

Bill had become a close friend too. I was finding out that being friends with all the groups was better than just being involved with one. So, I had Jock friends, and comedian friends. I also had a few "burnout" friends because of all the pot they smoked and just regular friends. I also had a lot of girls that were friends. I didn't want them to be friends, I wanted them in my bed. But most of the time I'd settle for a friendship that I hoped would blossom into more. They never did until I was thin. Then they came out of the woodwork. Having girls that are friends is really rare. If you are a good-looking girl and you think that all your guy friends are platonic, they're not thinking the same as you. They still want in your pants. It's high school. The hormone level is warp speed 5. Wake the hell up! They all want to sleep with you. That's just how guys are built. They'll play the friend zone game until you have that one night where you break down and cross the friend zone and pull one of those guys out. He'll give you the best sex you've ever had because that's all he's been thinking about for many years. You'll fall head over heels for him and then he'll dump you for putting him in the friend zone for so many years. More revenge against the pretty people of the world. I did it once, and I must say it felt kind of good. I had tried so many times to get this girl to see me as more than a friend. When she finally did, she was such a head case and I was the rebound boyfriend that when she called me up yelling at me about something I had never said, I hung up on her and didn't see her until the 20-year reunion. She jumped into my arms there, I guess she had forgotten all the shit she threw at me when we ended. I took that girl everywhere. We saw Elton John together; I took her out to dinner a couple of times a week. Blah. blah. Blah. If she ever reads this book, she'll know that it's her I'm talking about. To spend all that time not only trying to get her to see me but then getting her to take me out of the friend zone and become more than that was more of a nightmare than I ever thought it would be. Barb, you could have had me forever. That's how much I felt for you. But you put your faith in a guy who had dumped you for another woman who then lambasted me. Why couldn't you have believed me? I never lied to you, and you know Rick lied to you so many times it was painful for me to watch from my front-row seat. And by the way staying in line with the main subject of this book, the guy who made the most fun of me being fat in high school was Rick. He was a good friend at the time, so I let it slide. I wish I had it back. I would have never let him make fun of my weight in front of you or any other girl. But you went and believed his story and years later, you married the wrong guy too. At least after the way I saw him treat you at the reunion, he seemed like the wrong guy. He also posted something very nasty on my Facebook wall after the reunion. Nice guy. Hope you two are happy. I really do. Maybe you deserve one another. One other thing, Barb. Tim told me that he slept with you and so did Mike. So, I guess I was never good enough. You really missed out, let me tell you.

When the girls in high school saw me play hockey they usually were impressed. I was a goalie when we played rat hockey at the ice arena. I had been practicing with that college team I mentioned earlier and had gotten good. After some of the girls watched me play, they might snuggle up to me at Denny's after the game. I'd get compliments from them but then some asshole of a buddy would say "He's good because he takes up the whole net! No one can get anything past him because he's so fat." Suddenly, the girl wasn't sitting so close to me after that remark. I'd give the evil eye to my friend who said it and they'd go "What? What did I say? Usually, as I was pouring coffee all over their meal. These remarks may have been made in jest. But when you're the only one getting picked on because you're the fat guy it hurts bad. I wanted to have a girlfriend just as much as the next guy. When the opportunity presented itself, someone was always there to screw it up. I finally realized my senior year of high school, that if I was interested in someone, I had to get them alone with no interference from my so-called friends. So, I'd have to catch them between classes when we were alone with none of my stupid friends around. When this opportunity arose, I also had to make sure none of her friends were around. That way, I could find out whether or not she was interested in me and my personality or if she wasn't, then I would move on to the next candidate. My friend Bill D. found out that a girl in his neighborhood liked me. I didn't know this girl but when Bill said we should go on a double date I agreed faster than a new version of anything by Microsoft needing to be patched. Her name was Sherri and I found out she was a sophomore at school. That worked out for a little while until she dumped me, probably because someone gave her shit about the fat guy she was dating. And then later on during senior year a girl named Collen. We were together for about a month or so. When I started to get handsy, she started to get slappy. I finally got tired of it and gave up. I have one failed girl I have to tell you about. Melissa E. was one of the prettiest girls in school. She was incredibly shy, though. At least that's what I gathered on the information front. Every time I saw her eyes, I would think about robbing a bank to try to impress her with all the money I had. We didn't have a lot of classes together and didn't run in the same crowds, but I wanted just one shot at her. Just one moment when we were alone, and I could ask her out without people making fun of me because I was fat or her friends trying to convince her to say no because I was overweight. I never got that chance. Then she was just gone. She never went to the parties I was at, and I didn't even know if she had a boyfriend. At least that would have been a good excuse not to date me. So, wherever you are, Melissa, remember a fat guy who was chasing you around Tinley Park High School that wanted you so bad, and yet we could never get close enough to each other for me to ask you out. I know I wasn't pretty, but I would have treated you like a queen.

By the time I had gotten to the end of my senior year of high school, I was 290 pounds on a 6'2" frame. I am barrel-chested and have big shoulders. I didn't let being overweight slow me down. I played hard in gym class and usually surprised the gym teachers with my ability to do whatever we were doing. I tried hard not to let my extra weight stop me from doing athletic things. Some stuff I just wasn't good at. Like basketball. Too much running. But golf or dodgeball, look out. I was shooting in the low 90s during my senior year of high school. I even shot a couple of games in the mid-eighties.

We would have a competition at the end of each year to crown the class winner. The freshman would take on the juniors, and the sophomores against the seniors. The winners would take on each other for the championship. It was fun. We did everything from tricycle races to tug of war. I, being the largest boy in the senior class, was the anchor of the tug-of-war rope. These events were in front of the entire school. I was involved in at least three competitions. But the tug of war is the one I remember. I started the cadence to pull at the same time. We won the preliminary and the final. I finally felt like a leader. At that moment,

I had the most confidence I had ever had in high school. I wanted to ask every girl in the senior section out. You know, get a little black book and pencil girls in every day of the week. Yeah sure. Like that was going to happen. Just as I was leaving the area in front of the crowd, muscles tense and very visible I heard some girls say "Look at his arms!" I felt really good when I heard that. Then someone up high in the bleachers said, "way to go, fat Moss!" talk about bringing your confidence down. I didn't see who said it. I know it was a guy, but the only thing I could do was try to pretend I hadn't heard it. I did hear a lot of my senior class giggling. That pissed me off enough to try to find out who had said "way to go, fat Moss." I asked a bunch of people and no one knew who said it. I let it go even though it was probably in the top 3 embarrassing events that happened to me in high school.

Chapter 10

Before I move past the perils of high school for an overweight guy, I'd like to thank someone if she's still around. Her name was Mrs. Kirk. You see, we had to have 4 years of English in high school. The other English teachers made those classes pure torture for me because they wouldn't let me do creative writing the way I wanted to do it. I like to write like I talk and add humor to whatever I'm writing. Mrs. Kirk was the only one who would let me do that. I would right the wildest, funniest stories I could think of. She would correct my terrible spelling and grammar errors, but she didn't hold that against me. It might have dropped my grade from an A to an A- but that was it. She would always say that I needed to do something with my creative writing. Maybe work at a newspaper or write books or articles for magazines. I ended up choosing the first two. I wrote a newspaper column for 7 years just commenting on funny things that happen when you are raising 4 kids. I got a lot of compliments on it and eventually turned all the columns into two books. They are available on Amazon under Scott Moss books. There is also a novel there called Roadside. If you search Roadside by Scott Moss, you'll find it. Without Mrs. Kirk's advice and teaching skills in the back of my mind, the columns or books never would have happened. So, if she is still on this earth, someone shows her what a difference she made. She was a great teacher.

After graduation, I had saved for a trip to Disney World with my friend Jeff T. We were both making good money our senior year of high school, so we decided to buy the tickets to Orlando early in senior year. The plane tickets were for the week right after graduation. We both saved money to get into the park which I think was 25 dollars. It's about 160 dollars now. We stayed at a Marriott in Orlando, FL. We had gone to the park the first full day we were there. Now mind you I was still around 290 pounds. My friend Jeff was kind of a beanpole and was about 6'7" tall. The first thing we did when we got in the park was went into a gift shop and bought Mickey Mouse ears and start running from ride to ride. We were like little kids, trying to get as many rides in as possible. When we came up to one of the loop rollercoasters, they had a seat for the rollercoaster by the entrance. It was there to make sure you could fit on the ride before you waited in line. When I got in it the arm you pulled over your head wouldn't go all the way down so the bar would snap into the seatbelt. Pretty embarrassing. Jeff was trying to push the bar all the way down and we were only an inch from it snapping. I was gathering a crowd, all watching the fat guy trying to get in the seat. Someone came up to me and said they had seatbelt extenders at the end of the line. I got to ride the rollercoaster being the only one who needed an extender on the seatbelt. It was both fun and incredibly embarrassing. Thank God I didn't need to do that again for the rest of the time there that day. We stayed away from that coaster for the rest of the week.

The next day we slept in and when I met Jeff in the lobby, we decided to lie by the pool. I was laying on my stomach almost asleep when a girl started rubbing suntan lotion on my back. She did my whole back and even the back of my legs telling me the whole time about the suntan lotion. I thought to myself "why is a swimsuit model rubbing suntan lotion on my back when I weigh 290 pounds?" Another girl was doing the same thing to Jeff. I realized this was just a commercial for suntan lotion with live models. She wanted to do my front, but I didn't think that was a good idea. She looked like a supermodel, and I was an 18-year-old kid who was going to embarrass himself if I turned over. I just bought the bottle of lotion, and she disappeared in about three seconds. Pretty good sales campaign though. Got me to buy a bottle just because of the massage. Jeff bought one too. I thought I finally had a chance with a Coppertone girl, and it turns out she was just a salesperson for them. Damn it. Jeff and I drove go-carts that week. The first thing that was said to me when I got to the front of the line was that I might be too fat to get in a go-cart. I squeezed in that thing with very little difficulty. We ended up spending 150 dollars apiece driving this formula one-looking go-carts around a track to see who could get the best time. One hundred and fifty dollars was a lot of money to spend driving formula one go-carts in 1980. After doing that for about 3 hours we decided to go into this mom-and-pop diner that was on International drive. We got in and they only had booths. When I went to sit in the booth my stomach was right up against the table. The table was bolted to the floor, so I had to sit there and have a meal that felt like someone was giving me a bear hug around my stomach for the whole meal. There were a group of girls in the diner who kept looking over at me and giggling. Talk about embarrassing. I couldn't wait to get out of there. I ended up back in the hotel room feeling pretty down on myself. That's when I started to commit to losing weight. I can still see those 4 girls looking at me from their booth just like it was yesterday. But now, I'd like to thank them. They're part of the reason I started losing weight. Every time I got close to cheating on my diet I would flash back to those girls and put the treat back. Embarrassment is a pretty strong motivating factor during weight loss. It's another sad part of this journey.

So, let's move past high school now into work for me for a while. I had been working in the hospital in housekeeping. I worked full time most of my senior year of high school. I was making about between 300 to 400 dollars a week in 1980. To an 18-year-old, that was a shitload of money. I even bought a new Toyota Celica for myself. I was pretty sure I was the only senior who paid for his own new car. It seemed like a good idea at the time, but the insurance for an 18-year-old in a new car was astronomical. I only had the car for a little over a year, but a lot of pretty girls didn't mind riding around in a new car with a fat guy.

I worked in housekeeping for about 6 months. During that time, I started going to the gym with my friend Bill D. Bill never let me quit. Even though there were lots of times I wanted to, he wouldn't let me. My mom had read about Atkin's diet in a magazine article, so I bought the book. I had all morning to work out on most days. Bill and I would get to the gym at 6:00 am every morning except Sundays and work out for about an hour and a half. Cardio wasn't a thing back then. It was all weight machines and free weights. I don't ever remember seeing a treadmill in the entire place for the two years I went there. Bill kept me on this regime until all the weight was gone. We would go out to breakfast and because I could only have meat, eggs, cheese, and coffee, so I always had an omelet. (I'm sure there were more foods, but those are the ones I spent the most time eating) I also ate carrots or celery with cheese on it as a snack. I lost about 90 pounds in about six months. About halfway through the weight loss program, some of the girls at the hospital were starting to look at me as more than a friend. A girl I worked with in physical therapy as an aide had been on my radar since she started. I was pretty sure she was the same age as me. She was so shy she barely spoke. I tried to get her to laugh and open up to me. She had shorter black hair and the most beautiful green eyes I had ever seen up until that point in my life. I was about halfway or so to my weight loss goal, so I decided to give it a chance and ask her out. When she said yes, I almost fell over. She was so beautiful I didn't think she'd say yes. But I sure wasn't going to look a gift horse in the mouth. I have to stop here for a second. What the hell does that saying mean? My dad used to say it and he was born in 1931 so maybe I got it from him and he's long past, so I still have no idea what it means. Anyhow back to our story. The first time I went to Kim's house to pick her up for a date her ex-husband came out to greet me. Kim had a 2-year-old daughter, so I guess he was there to see her. I thought he might be looking for a fight, so I quickly got out of my car. Kim was on the front porch with a mortified look on her face. The guy introduced himself as Kim's ex-husband and that he was there to see his daughter. No threats or anything. He was actually kind of nice. Maybe my size was a little intimidating. He was a smaller guy but never seemed to be a threat. Kim did have some explaining to do. Not only did I not know about the ex-husband, but I also didn't know about the baby. I asked her about all of this after we pulled out of the driveway. When I asked her about it, she said "I didn't want you to think that I was loose from having a baby and being married at a young age." This is the most she's ever said to me in one sentence. I said "do you think that would matter to me? Because it doesn't. I love kids so I can't wait to see her. As for the loose thing, I do know a little about anatomy and what happens after childbirth. So, if you're referring to what I think you are referring to, I'm not worried." I think she thought it would matter to me that she had a child. She was a very young mother. Probably at 17 or less. She was from the south hence the early marriage. They had been divorced for over a year and she said he's only come up to see the baby a few times. She was staying in the main floor bedroom of her parent's house while her parents slept upstairs. We had a lot of fun in that bedroom. We lasted about 3 months until she found someone else. I went right for that guy's old girlfriend and as payback. She spent some seriously fun time with me. I think he was approached by her, so I obviously wasn't the end game.

I purposely stayed away from some of the parties at my friends from high school houses. I wanted to lose all of it before I went. Most of the time I was working anyhow, so it wasn't a big deal. When I got down to 210 pounds and had reached my goal of losing 90 pounds, Bill and I went to this party at a girl's house that we graduated with. There were a lot of people there. A lot of girls too. Most of them never gave me a look. Now Bill and I were both big by now. The only problem we had was that if Bill had a little too much to drink, he liked to fight. So in between talking to girls who hadn't seen me in 6 months and keeping Bill from beating the crap out of some guy for spilling beer on his shoe, it was lots of fun. Girls that never talked to me throughout high school were suddenly giving me compliments and sitting close to me on the couch. I was now working full-time days in a physical therapy department so I could go out more. I started dating girls like crazy. I was always nice, and every girl got treated to dinner or a movie and then maybe some ice cream. Wherever it went from there was completely up to them. I never pushed anyone for sex. I let it happen when it was supposed to. It's different for each woman.

There was one girl I had always wanted. I mentioned her before in this book but at this point, she needs to be mentioned again. Barb was a girl I followed around the school like a puppy dog for all four years. We had become friends by junior year, but it wasn't till senior year that we got close. Unfortunately, she was dating my best friend for most of my senior year. Just after graduation, Rick broke up with Barb for a blond with a big mouth and the willingness to do anything with him. And when I say anything, I mean anything. I did not like this girl at all. She would twist people's words around to make herself look better and ended up causing a lifetime friendship to end. She told Rick I said I was going to kick his ass if I got in the way of Barb and me. Something I never said.

After I lost all the weight, I wanted Barb. Everyone else was playing second fiddle. She was it for me. Or so I thought. I had lost all the weight by now and had a Friday night where I had nothing planned for a change. I was going to sit at home and relax. My mom told me Barb was on the phone. She was still a mess from the breakup, so I knew she just wanted to vent with me. 30 minutes later 5 girls showed up at my door. Barb was one of them and the rest were mutual friends of ours. Two of them hadn't seen me since I lost weight, so I got to see that reaction. It was always fun for me to stand up and hug them so they could feel how thin and muscular I was. I know, I was a little full of myself back then. Some of them wanted to stay to talk to me but my friend Betty got them all out of there. They left me with Barb. We sat on the couch in my basement, and I let her tell her sob story again to me. I saw Rick over the years take advantage of girls right and left. She was just the last one on the list at that time. She wanted him back. I wanted her to shut up about it and be with me. Finally, that night, Barb was sitting right next to me on the couch with her head on my shoulder still shedding tears. I picked up her chin and decided it was time to stop this. I brought my lips down on hers and laid the biggest, deepest, most passionate kiss on her that I could. She went with it and kissed me right back. We spent the next two hours making out on the couch and started to explore each other a little bit. This kept going on either in the car or at her house or mine. A lot of time was spent in her driveway too. I was falling hard for this girl. I mean big-time hard. I should have got a clue about her personality when she wouldn't go out with me until I lost the weight. If she had been whom I thought she was, the weight wouldn't have mattered. But at the time, I was just happy to be with her.

After a couple of months, we were starting to get closer, and I wanted to go away for a weekend with her. The week I had made the reservation we were in her driveway on a Wednesday night. We were making out, laying on the front seat. Rick pulled up behind me and put his bright lights on. We sat up and I said, "who the fuck is that?" I should have known because he had an old galaxy 500 that his dad and him fixed up. It had loud pipes on it. By the time I heard those, I knew it was him. He came up to my window and said "Bud, we have to talk." then got back in his car and pulled up to the front of Barb's garage, and shut his car off. Barb didn't say anything to me. She just jumped out of my car and got right into his. I now knew what a rebound guy was. I was crushed. I spent all that time and put all that work in to lose all that weight to hopefully date my dream girl someday and the moment her old boyfriend shows up, she drops me faster than a toupee in a hurricane. Needless to say, I canceled the weekend in Lake Geneva, Wisconsin the next day. I found out later on that Terri had started the rumor that I was telling everyone about Barb and I being together and that if Rick tried to get in the way, I was going to kick his ass. The next time I heard from Barb was when she was yelling at me saying that I was telling everyone that she was my girlfriend. I hadn't told anyone what we were doing. Rick's new girlfriend who would later become his wife and then his ex-wife who took him for everything because the guy she was cheating with was a divorce lawyer and Rick couldn't afford a good one. Unfortunately, there were two beautiful little girls in the mix of that disaster. Even after all that shit, I still feel sorry for what he went through with that bitch. She took away the ability for him to see his girls every day. She took most of his money, and did I mention she was a bitch?

What does any of this have to do with my weight journey? It has a lot to do with it. I thought that if I lost all the weight, I would have the girl of my dreams. Turned out, she ended up being a nightmare at that time. We've since made up and other than me not being able to tolerate her husband, she's back to what I'd consider a friend although she lives halfway across the country in the state I'd like to retire to. I'm not talking about God's waiting room in Florida. She's in Colorado and I've always wanted to have a summer home there. I have no desire to be there in the winter, I'll rent the place out. But Colorado is beautiful in the summer. No humidity either like we have in the Midwest. We had reunions when I got to see her. On the thirtieth-year reunion, the music was so loud I couldn't hear her. We had a karaoke party, and most people didn't know that I could sing. I must have sung eight songs. I wowed the crowd and so did my friend Dean H. Dean was one of the funniest guys and had the sweetest girlfriend in the world. Dean and Laurie are still friends today. My wife and I go out to dinner with them every once in a while. Dean would sing country songs and I would sing classic rock songs. Not too many others participated but we would drag people up there and make them sing back up or if we could talk them into singing a song, they would. It wasn't a big crowd, but it sure was fun. When I tried to talk to Barb during the reunion it was very hard to hear her. She was a soft talker, and I just couldn't communicate with her. I got her phone number and called her the next day. The next Friday, I took her out to breakfast at a great bakery by her house. Yes, I got permission from my wife. I just needed to get some questions answered. That's all I was interested in. I was way back up in weight by this time in my life and she was still beautiful at 50 or so. I just wanted to see what her take was on the nasty phone call she gave me that completely trashed our relationship. I wondered about that for 30 years. All that anger still floating around in my veins and what does she say when I brought the whole thing up? She said she didn't remember yelling at me. She couldn't believe she would do something like that to me. I told her I remembered it like it was yesterday. To her, it wasn't in the least bit important. To me, it meant everything. Shows you how you can be so excited about someone, and they are just using you as a rebound guy. I learned a valuable lesson that day. Mainly to let a lot of stuff go. I remember so much that it sometimes causes me problems. Especially when it comes to all the people in my past who made fun of me for being heavy. I'm a little too sensitive and have been all my life. It started with my parents being hard on us to the things that happened a little over a year ago. I can forgive but I never forget. That can be a pretty hard way to live. Being overweight played right into those insecurities. I found out I fit the description of what is called an empath. Look it up, you'll find it very interesting. I have the ability to feel other peoples moods. So being around a bunch of angry or depressed people isn't good. You know that one friend who always knows when you are in a bad mood before you say anything? That's me. Read a little bit about it. It's very interesting. No I'm not crazy.

Chapter 11

The hospital

After the debacle with Barb, I decided I was only going to ask out girls from the hospital. I had a 250-bed hospital with a nurse for every 4 beds. And three shifts of them. I never saw the night nurses, but the days and 3 to 11-shift nurses were all fair game for me. I loved being in great shape. I felt like I had so much more energy. I was still not as confident as I should have been but being shot down by so many girls when I was in high school, so I was still a little gun shy. I always dated one girl at a time. I wasn't a man whore. I was very careful not to fall back into old habits. I was drinking one glass of milk a day. No more than that. I still stuck to the meat, eggs, and cheese following the basics of the diet. I was now having salads too. Anything healthy. I was still going to the gym about 4 days a week. I was also lifting 250-pound stroke patients in and out of bed. My main job was transporting patients to and from the physical therapy department. Sometimes up to 30 trips a day. At times when we were really busy, I could push two wheelchairs at once to make things move faster in the department. I was on my feet running most of the time. But the nice thing about this job was I got to see nurses from every floor in the hospital. If one of them caught my eye, I would make sure I took all the patients from that floor up there and made sure I got a chance to talk to the nurse in question. My confidence was up higher, and I wasn't afraid to ask any nurse or tech, or physical therapist out. I even asked a doctor out. She was nice. We had two very nice dates. She was in the process of either going out with her boyfriend or being broken up with him. I was a distraction when she was away from her boyfriend. She was a sweetheart. I think she was getting back at him through me, and I wasn't complaining at all.

One of the problems with being young and having too much money at that time was the fact that I looked old enough to buy beer. Beer isn't good for a low-carb diet. Beer is loaded with it. But I'm not a mixed drink person. I stuck to beer. I had to work hard in the gym to keep from gaining weight back. I drank too much on the weekend but nothing during the week. I was too committed to work to drink during the week. I liked what I did. Although working with doctors can drive you completely crazy. Back then they thought that the world revolved around them. Nobody policed them. They got away with more shit than you would ever believe. There were some good ones too. I just tried to stay out of their way. Besides, I had a real life now that I was thin. People didn't make fun of me. Everyone who hadn't seen me since I lost all the weight couldn't believe what I looked like now. It was so nice. But I didn't give some people the time of day. Mainly the ones that made fun of me when I was fat. Especially the girls. I had a few of them make moves on me and I ignored them. It was a lot of fun. I couldn't believe that someone who was so mean to me could turn around and act like it didn't matter that I should feel special and that they wanted to go out with me. I worked so hard to get to this ideal weight and I wasn't going to waste time on people who thought it was ok to make fun of me.

Being overweight for a long time is just like an addiction. Just substitute sugar for alcohol. You may think that it's all a matter of controlling your urges. But what's funny is people who are addicted to alcohol and drugs are a small percentage of people compared to the obesity problem in the United States. Obesity in children has increased by a huge amount since video games became the main entertainment for children. Let's look at some of the numbers:

Nationally, **41.9 percent** of adults are obese. Black adults had the highest level of adult obesity at 49.9 percent. Hispanic adults had an obesity rate of 45.6 percent. Obesity is defined by first finding out what your BMI is. There are calculators all over the internet. You plug in your height and weight, and it will give you your BMI. If it's over 30 you are considered obese. Not overweight, obese. Being obese is dangerous for so many reasons. You can acquire high blood pressure. Also, type two diabetes. A hazardous disease that can do everything from having an early heart attack to losing circulation in your legs. Many long-term type II diabetics end up as amputees. Obesity is at epidemic proportions in this country. It's killing people every day. Now let's look at childhood obesity:

As of 2020[2], 19.7% of all children and teens in the US were obese. I'm sure that number is at 20% by now because of kids being locked up at home because of covid. Black and Hispanic children have disproportionately represented in this number: 26.2% of Hispanic and 24.8% of Black children were obese, compared with 16.6% of non-Hispanic White and 9.0% of non-Hispanic Asian children. Children in low-income households are also likelier to be obese.

So at least two out of ten children are obese. Not overweight, obese. That's scary. There is a category after obesity called morbid

---

2. https://www.cdc.gov/obesity/data/childhood.html#_853ae90f0351324bd73ea615e6487517__4c761f170e016836ff84498202b99827__853ae90f0351324bd73ea615e6487517_text_43ec3e5dee6e706af7766fffea512721_Prevalence_0bcef9c45bd8a48eda1b26eb0c61c869_20of_0bcef9c45bd8a48eda1b26eb0c61c869_20Childhood_0bcef9c45bd8a48eda1b26eb0c61c869_20Obesity_0bcef9c45bd8a48eda1b26eb0c61c869_20in_0bcef9c45bd8a48eda1b26eb0c61c869_20the_0bcef9c45bd8a48eda1b26eb0c61c869_20United_0bcef9c45bd8a48eda1b26eb0c61c869_20States_6cff047854f19ac2aa52aac51bf3af4a_text_43ec3e5dee6e706af7766fffea512721_For_0bcef9c45bd8a48eda1b26eb0c61c869_20children_0bcef9c45bd8a48eda1b26eb0c61c869_20and_0bcef9c45bd8a48eda1b26eb0c61c869_20adolescents_0bcef9c45bd8a48eda1b26eb0c61c869_20aged_c0cb5f0fcf239ab3d9c1fcd31fff1efc_14.7_0bcef9c45bd8a48eda1b26eb0c61c869_20million_0bcef9c45bd8a48eda1b26eb0c61c869_20children_0bcef9c45bd8a48eda1b26eb0c61c869_20and_0bcef9c45bd8a48eda1b26eb0c61c869_20adolescents

obesity. These people have trouble even walking. Morbid obesity has become so prevalent that at least 5 people you'll see per day are morbidly obese. That's just my estimate. I know what it's like to be that way because I was there for years. 1 in 4 (24.2%) will be considered severely obese by 2030. For a patient to be considered clinically severe, or morbidly obese, he or she must have a **body mass index or BMI of 35–39.9 with one or more severe health conditions or a BMI of 40 or greater**. Again, look up the BMI calculator and plug in your height and weight and you'll get your BMI when you refer to the chart that goes with the BMI calculator. At my heaviest, during my lifetime I had a BMI of 49.4. That is morbidly obese with a capital M.

My highest BMI which occurred at about the age of 58 was 49.4. That is ridiculous. I'll get to that in a little while. Stay tuned.

Chapter 12

Think first, pay later

As I decided not to focus on my old high school girls, I started dating the nurses at the hospital. I found out that being a 19-year-old who looks like a 23-year-old made it easy to get a couple of drinks at the bar. So, when I took one of the nurses out, I didn't tell them how old I really was until I decided if the relationship was worth continuing. I didn't always get a good vibe from a date. I went out with this girl who worked with me in the vascular lab at the hospital. She was a beautiful blond-haired girl with the most beautiful body. Unfortunately, from the time I picked her up till the time I dropped her off, she talked excessively. I'm not sure I even got to say hello. The next date was better, but we were still having trouble communicating. We went to a carnival with my friend Mike and his date. Mike worked at the hospital with me too. He was in housekeeping, and we went to parties a lot together. We even went to a completely insane toga party thrown by the emergency room department that was so much fun I have never forgotten it. At that party, I noticed that Mike and Sherri were talking a lot and getting along well. I could tell he liked her a lot. She didn't seem to be that interested in me. Mike came up to me during the party and asked if it would be ok if he took Sherri home. I had my eye on someone else at the party, so I told Mike to go ahead, she doesn't seem interested in me anyway. They ended up going out for over a year. I made out with the girl I had my eye on at the party. I got her number and we all ended up in a conga line completely covered in beer. Thank God we didn't get stopped by the cops that night. It smelled like a brewery in my car that night. I was glad that luck was on our side, and nothing happened. We were pretty stupid back then and didn't think that much about drinking and driving. I wouldn't allow anyone to drink in my car while we were going somewhere. I didn't want a ticket or to go sit in a jail cell because my idiot friends wanted to start partying early. But still, we could have been killed so many times. I mentioned my friend Jimbo earlier in this book. When we were 17, he moved down to Arizona with his family. A drunk semi-truck driver blew a stop sign and killed Jim instantly. I remember getting that call and being in shock for days. I had been friends with him since we were 6. I was a little more careful about drinking and driving from that point on. I wasn't perfect, but I did watch how much I drank when I was driving. Sorry, off on another tangent again. I realize this is more of an autobiography of a fat guy than anything else. I hope you don't mind me telling some stories about my weight loss and gain story. I want the book to be fun to read rather than just another diet book. That's not what this is. It's a book about the life of a man who struggled with a significant weight problem. But stories keep a book interesting. That's why I'm going with them in this book. Try to keep up.

 I had been maintaining the goal weight of between 210 and 220 for about a year when we got a new bunch of physical therapists in the department. It was always so weird. They would come and go in threes or fours. Of the first four, I worked with 2 of them moved on to different hospitals for more money. The third one was a girl named Gail. She wasn't there very long but she was so beautiful I had a hard time concentrating while she was around. Gail was a natural blond with the most hypnotizing blue eyes I had ever seen. They were bright blue. I would talk to her about a patient and trail off because I was staring into her eyes so much. I really was hoping I could somehow get to her and see if she would have a little fling or even more before she got married. She was engaged shortly after she started. But she was truly in love, and you could tell. Even flirting with her didn't faze her. I admired her because she had fallen deeply in love and didn't want to risk it. I tried, I was so attracted to her that if I never had tried, I would regret it forever. When she was engaged, she was impenetrable. She loved her fiancé. So, I gave up the effort and she left the hospital before she got married. The third one became one of my best friends. He ended up moving out to Southern California. Because we had been so close as friends, I ended up using any vacation time I accrued to go out and see him. He lived 5 minutes from the beach. I would fly out there and sleep on his couch for a week while we saw the sites, went surfing, skied in the San Bernadino mountains, and tried to pick up any girl in a bikini. I wasn't embarrassed for the first time in my life to take my shirt off at the beach. I had finally reached the point were I could take my shirt off and not be embarrassed by the way I looked. My weight had stabilized at about 210 pounds. When I was in high school and my friend Rick would have a pool party, I would always wear a shirt in the pool to help cover up my fat body. This time out in California was the first time I didn't worry about being bare-chested. It's little things like that that will make you happy. Having girls look at me for a change was nice too. That was a completely different experience for me. Rich and I would meet a couple of girls on the beach and take them out that night. Both of us were single and took advantage of that status. I couldn't believe girls were asking me to come back home to their apartment after dinner and dancing. Rich never went home alone either. Remember, this was the early 1980s. No one worried about AIDS or even VD. It was a free for all kind of time. I picked the perfect time to be thin for that reason alone. We were still careful, but no one had the worries that they had later in the decade. Although there were a lot of nights where we would just go to the beach and watch the sunset while drinking some beer. It was one of the happiest periods of my life.

Rich's place in Southern California lost a lot of its luster after I brought one of the physical therapists I had fallen in love with out there. Then it became the place I lost her. She went back to her fiancé after sneaking around with me for six months. Her name was Kathy, and she was my first true love. I've only had my heart truly shattered once, and she was the one that did it. If she had said yes, we would have come home married. A small ceremony on the beach would have been just fine. We could have a reception when we got back home. Instead, she left a day early telling me she couldn't do this anymore. I got to watch her walk down the ramp at the airport and get on a plane to go directly out of my life. I could barely look at her when we got back to work on Monday. I was so mad at her for leading me on like that. I can take a lot of the blame, but she was the one that kissed me after we were the last ones to leave the bar one night. I had picked her up to play racquetball. Something we had been doing for months. We also played a lot of golf together too. That night after playing racquetball, we ended up having dinner and then went dancing at this little bar. When we left, I opened the door of the car for her, and she looked up at me and said, "my fiancé never opens the car door for me." I said, "If you pick me, I'll open the door for you for the rest of your life." When I came around and sat down in the driver's seat, I wanted to kiss her on the cheek just to let her know what a fun night I had with her. Everything up until that time had been platonic. As I went in for the kiss, she turned her head on purpose and I kissed her right on the lips. She then wrapped her hands around my neck and pulled me in for a very deep, passionate kiss. When we broke the kiss, I rested my forehead on hers and said, "do you know how long I've been waiting for that to happen?" she said shut up and recline the seats. I did just that and we had a really good time in the parking lot (yes, I moved the car to an empty part of the lot) kissing and feeling each other, starting something very special to me. That started a 6-month affair with her and me sneaking around almost every weeknight. She would have to see her fiancé on the weekends because he was still in school. Every once in a while, he would go motorcycle riding with his buddies, and I would get to take her away for the weekend. I think her brother knew about the affair and would cover for us. We tried to sneak away as often as possible. I tried so hard to get her to leave him, but I was so in love with her that I let her get away with staying engaged to him while she was with me. At the end of our relationship, we went to Las Vegas and then drove to California to stay with Rich. He was gone on a camping trip with his girlfriend for 3 days, so we had the place to ourselves. I think we christened every flat surface in that apartment in those three days. When Rich came back, he would close the door to his bedroom at night and we would make love every night too. Until she finally came to me in tears and said "I'm feeling so guilty, Scott. I can't do this anymore." the next day, she insisted on leaving. I put her on a plane a day early and she was gone. Like I said I was so mad at her that we barely talked for 3 weeks. Within a couple of days of getting back, I started to date other women immediately. They would come down and visit me in the department and I'd sneak them back into the conference room and make out with them for a couple of minutes before they went back upstairs. I wasn't really that interested in these women, I just wanted to make Kathy mad. Well, Kathy saw this a couple of times with different women and got really jealous. She finally confronted me about it. She just said, "can you meet me at our Ice Cream Shop right after work today?" I said "now why would I want to do that after the way you treated me?" She finally begged me, and I said I would. When we got to the ice cream shop and sat down outside, she actually had the nerve to ask me not to have so many girls come down to see me because she was getting really jealous. What I should have done next was pull her close to me and lay the biggest kiss on her in hopes of getting her back. What I did was tell her I can't be with her if she didn't give up that ring. I still wonder to this day if I had just kissed her and started the entire thing up again that I could have finally got her to leave him. She was so confused I almost felt sorry for her. I think she originally wanted a one-night affair with me but after we made love, she wanted 6 months of that. I still pursued her to a certain point after we got back and had our little talk 3 weeks later. I wasn't talking to her very much in the beginning, but I still helped her at work. I didn't make a big effort to go upstairs to work with her on patients, though. It was hard to be alone with her and not want to have her in my arms.

We used to kiss in the elevator a lot. We would get in the elevator right by physical therapy and as soon as the doors closed, we would start kissing like our lives depended on it. I wanted to try that again after she left me but never did. There was a part of me that was still so mad at her. But the part of me that wanted her back was strong. She bent her own rules a couple of times, kissing me but would never take it past that again. One of the physical therapy assistants named Joy S. had known about the affair from the beginning and kept warning me that I was going to get my heart broken. She said to me one day that I had to let her go. She said that Kathy wasn't strong enough to break things off with her fiancé so after weeks of Joy telling me I had to let her go I finally agreed with her.

Kathy was in the break room alone. When I saw her there, I went in and closed the door. She looked up at me and I said, "come here, please." She walked over to me, and I said "are you sure that you want to marry him instead of me? She looked down at her feet and then back up to me. With teary eyes, she said "I have to, Scott. He's been my life for 3 years. He loves me and I know that I can't hurt him." I said "you don't seem to have a problem hurting me though. Why is that? I love you more than anyone could love someone else." Now I was getting teary-eyed. I said "I want something from you right now, then I'll give you what you want. I need to kiss you one more time." She didn't hesitate. She came to my arms, and I put my hands on her cheeks and gave her everything I had in that kiss. I held her tight and finally said, "I'm going to let you go. It's the last thing I want to do but if it will make you happy, I'll do it." She hugged me again and by now tears had started to run down her face. Her wedding was in 6 weeks. It was the hardest thing I ever had to do. But after that, we went our separate ways.

Because I missed the wedding and the reception (I couldn't bare being in that church or reception hall without saying something) I didn't see her until after her honeymoon. He took her to Hawaii. I had the feeling the reason why she left me was that I didn't make enough money. She was right at first, he definitely made a lot more money than me and I think his family had money. I think (and this is just my opinion) she didn't want to struggle in the first couple of years of our marriage because I was going back to school, and we would have to live off of her salary and whatever I could make while I was in school. My cardiology program was only a year long, so it wouldn't have been a struggle forever. Her fiancé bought her a house right away and probably started his first job at 65,000 dollars a year. That was a lot of money in 1984. She told me once that money didn't matter to her but in the long run, it really did. If she had just had some faith in me I would have proven to her that I could be an excellent provider. For 30 years I made a 6-figure income. Maybe not as much as him, but still enough to make a good life together. But who's to say that things would have worked out that way? In the next chapter, you'll see how I was inspired to do better by someone else. Someone who taught me that true love shouldn't be as hard as it was with Kathy.

She went ahead with the wedding. When she sent me an invitation to the wedding, I put a big fat zero on the return card. She confronted me about it and all I said was "If you think I'm going to go to your wedding and watch you walk down the aisle with the wrong guy you're crazy. You know you should be with me, but you didn't have the guts to break it off with him." I did sit out in front of the church that day to see if she maybe would come running out of the church because she changed her mind, but of course, that only happens in the movies. She stayed married to him for a long time. But as you'll find out, everything happens for a reason.

Kathy passed away from cancer about a year ago as I was writing this book. There were a lot of things I wish I could have gotten answers to before she died. Unfortunately, I didn't know she was dying until she was already unconscious and, on her way out. She had become very religious, so I hope that got her to heaven and that I'll get to see her again. Although, I think I might have to spend some time in purgatory before that happens. I hope she has found peace. She suffered a lot from colon cancer. She had become a doctor and was loved by all her patients. She will always be the first girl I ever loved. Losing her before I got some answers to some very important questions that had come up years later would have been nice.

Chapter 13

My real love

I enjoyed being single for about 5 years after I lost the weight. The struggle never ended. I swear it's like alcohol but in the form of a snickers bar. They put them right by the checkout for a reason. They're for fat guys like me to pick up on the way out of the store. I'd go to Home Depot for 6 2x4s and come home with the 6 2x4s and 2 snickers bars. Always having to monitor what you eat isn't easy. Especially if you come from a family like mine where cooking good food is a way of life. We always had a family dinner on Sunday. If I had been dating someone for a month or so I would bring her to the festivities and afterward I would say "do you see why I had such a weight problem?" The girl would be holding her stomach because she ate so much thanks to my mother walking around the table and putting more food on everyone's plate. My girlfriend would say "she's awfully hard to say no to, isn't she?" It made my weight problem a little bit easier to understand.

Girls post-Kathy included one of the other physical therapists with whom I was great friends. One-night things got a little out of hand and we ended up on the living room floor with no clothes on. I would give you her name, but she might have me assassinated. I liked this girl. She was sweet and loving. She also came from a big family where her mom could put out quite a spread of food. I had dinner down there on her parent's farm several times. Her dad even let me drive the front-loading tractor. I got to move some gravel and it was better than any Tonka Truck I ever had. We dated for a while. We eventually figured out that we were better as friends than as lovers. She is still my friend today. I don't get to see her as much as I'd like to, but it's hard to get together with family and grandkids for both of us.

A month before I started the affair with Kathy, I started dating a girl named Eileen. She was this absolutely gorgeous, petite woman that was a nurse on one of the floors in the hospital. Because Kathy had yet to present herself as a lover, I kept dating other women. I was waiting to see if Kathy would ever leave her fiancé for me. Because we had been getting closer and closer to each other I could sense something was coming. I was leaning toward just pulling her into me and kissing the snot out of her and see if I got her to kiss me back or if I was going to get slapped. But that day was a ways away. I asked Eileen out after we had talked a lot on the floor where she was working. When I finally got the nerve to ask her out, she said yes. I always loved petite women, and Eileen was one of them. All of 5'2" and 110 pounds she was so pretty I didn't think she would go out with me because she had been going out with the same guy for six years. Since high school. He had cheated on her a couple of times, and she wasn't happy about it. When I asked her out, she disposed of him faster than a cupcake at a weight watchers convention. We dated for a very hot month where we couldn't keep our hands off each other. She worked the 3 to 11 shift so we couldn't be together all the time. When we could go out the date always ended up tangled in each other's arms. There was something about this girl. But I had no desire at that time to settle down. I had 4 years of high school to make up for and a little bit more. But this one made me think. She scared me. Her family was so fun and the parties she threw at her condo were over the top. I was going over to her house on a Wednesday for her birthday. On Tuesday, Kathy finally attacked me after we left a bar. Engagement ring and all. I had waited for over a year for this to happen. I just kept trying to get closer to her every day I worked with her. Trying to make her laugh and being with her when we played on the golf league, the bowling team, and racquetball. Whenever we golfed together, I would purposely hit my ball near hers just so we could talk more. We drank a lot of beer and by the end of the nine-hole game, we were laughing pretty hard at each other. The same was true with bowling. All these sports were generated by someone making up a league from the hospital. I knew the person who made up the golf league. I asked him a favor to pair me with Kathy for every round. He said, "Isn't she engaged?" I said, "Yes. But I'm hoping that she won't be soon." He wanted to help so he set me up with her. The bowling league was department tournaments. So, we'd play respiratory therapy one week and then the team from housekeeping the next. It was perfect for a bunch of young 20-something groups to have a lot of fun.

After the attack (I like to call it that now because it was an all-out assault on my person) I realized I finally had gotten what I wanted. Kathy's undivided attention. We spent every possible moment together. Which meant I screwed things up with Eileen royally. I didn't even call her to tell her what happened and that I needed to see this thing with Kathy through. I was an idiot. For 2 main reasons. I bought into the absolute lie that Kathy would leave her fiancé and I completely screwed up things with Eileen. I hope she wasn't going to have me killed. She had a lot of brothers, so there was a chance. Turns out, she needed that time away from everyone including her old boyfriend. I spent 6 months trying to get the girl of my dreams (or so I thought) to leave her fiancé. I told you about our trip together and how she put an end to our relationship. I was a wreck for several months after that happened. I had a real good thing going with Eileen and I was sure she wouldn't forgive me. I went on a warpath for a while going to bars to see if I could pick up anything with a pulse and go back to their apartment with them. Mine or hers, it didn't matter. Nameless, faceless women to try to forget the face of the one woman I thought I couldn't live without. This was the early 80s, so I got pretty lucky to not end up with a disease.

Then something happened that I never expected. Eileen's mother passed away. My mom kept bugging me to make an appearance at the wake. I felt like this wasn't a good idea because she was probably still furious with me. But my mom could be pretty persuasive at the time and had her black belt in guilt, I took a chance and showed up there hoping she wouldn't throw me out. She did just the opposite. She was happy to see me. I said that I was sorry for her loss and apologized for how things had ended between us promising to tell her why if she would let me take her out again. My kids make fun of me for catching her at a weak moment. I had a little more tack than that, but I guess I saw an opportunity once I realized she wasn't going to have me killed, I pulled her to the side and asked her if she would give me another chance. She said she would. The following week we went out again and I got a chance to explain the whole Kathy saga to her. She understood why I did what I did. She just wished I had called her to let her know what was going on. She was pretty hurt, and I can never get that back. But I've been trying to make it up to her for the last 39 years. She was the real deal. The one person I think God put on this earth for me. She has been through hell and back with me. Especially putting up with my weight gain that came approximately 15 to 20 minutes after we got married.

Chapter 14

The roller coaster

I was 22 when I got married. Eileen was 24. I always kid her about robbing the cradle. We had a beautiful wedding at a well know reception hall just south of Chicago. The place was called The Martinique. There were 300 people there. About 150 of them were just extended family and the rest were friends we both had become close to. We all had so much fun. Dancing and talking to people I hadn't seen in so long. I felt it was safe now to invite Kathy to the wedding because we had been such good friends before any of the passion. I had planned to sing to Eileen during the reception. I sang a song called "She's got a way" by Billy Joel. It seemed to be written for Eileen. Look up the lyrics of the song and picture a guy with a bad 80s haircut in a white tux to show my purity and innocence. (Insert laughter here). About halfway through the song I looked up and met eyes with Kathy. I looked at her and she got up quickly and made a beeline for the bathroom. She had a tissue in her hand. Eileen's sisters had brought her up on stage so I could sing directly to her. It was about as romantic as I could be. After the song was over, I kissed Eileen and then had my brother Tim come up on stage with me and because I had the white tux on, I decided to sing "Ice Cream Man" by Van Halen. My brother Tim acted out all of David Lee Roth's jumps and I sang my ass off. I got a standing ovation and as I stepped off stage I looked over at Kathy and she was just sitting in her seat looking down. I didn't think too much about it until it was time for the end of the reception. I was saying by to a lot of people. As I was about to walk out Kathy was standing in front of me. In a very timid voice, she said "we're going to go" I said, "Kathy, this could have all been for you. Every minute of it. You know that don't you?" she nodded her head. I leaned forward and kissed her on the cheek. She hugged me and I could hear her sniffling. Then she walked away quickly. Maybe someone was second-guessing her decision? I really hoped she was. She crushed me so a little revenge would have been appropriate. I watched her leave, knowing I might never see her again when that saying popped into my mind "Everything happens for a reason." I met Eileen in the middle of the dance floor, and we went to a party at my parent's house. We had an afternoon reception, so it ended at about 5:00. Eileen and I made a stop at my parent's house to change, and off we were for our two-day honeymoon. I was starting school on Tuesday. We went to a resort in the northern suburbs of Chicago. It wasn't a long honeymoon, but we had planned to see San Diego after I was done with school. It was a wonderful couple of days, we even went golfing between jumping each other's bones in the hotel room.

    I hadn't gone to college like a lot of people back then. My parents didn't have the money for me to go to college and I hated the idea of going to 4 years of school to get to the last year to finally learn what you needed to become an accountant or a business specialist. I needed a crash course in a career that required an on-the-job type of training. A fantastic doctor I knew named Doctor Branit helped me get into a vocational school at a different hospital that was training Cardio-Vascular specialists. We went to school 5 days a week for 8 hours a day. We learned all the testing in cardiology. I would sometimes have 4 hours of homework every night. I quit my job at the hospital right after Eileen and I were married. The very next week I started school. We wear living off of one income for the first three months. I gained about 25 pounds back because I was so sitting on my ass all day just watching technologists do testing and learning how to work the machines. Then having to do 4 hours of homework every night. I finished the program in a year. During that time, I was a bouncer at a rather large bar to help make some extra money for our new life. The night someone pulled a very large knife on me was the night I quit that job and started working weekend nights as a print shop photographer. I was the guy responsible for sizing pictures so they would fit in the right spots in the newspaper. A pretty mindless job but it paid better than the possibility of being stabbed.

When I started school, I was still thin. I was one of 12 students. 3 of us were guys. So, we were all outnumbered. I got some looks from a couple of girls in the class but when they saw the wedding ring it stopped them. All but one of them. She would touch my arm and rub up against me during our class picture at the beginning of the year. She was pretty, but I was content and happy. But just so you know, it's not always the married guy trying to pick up a woman.

About 4 months in I had gained about 25 pounds. My stomach was back, and my muscle tone was fading. I had no time for working out. I was either in school, studying, or working all week. Eileen never said anything mean to me about gaining the weight back. I was hoping to put a stop to it once we were done with the anatomy and physiology part of the classroom work, but I had already fallen back into old habits. I started drinking milk again. I couldn't seem to stay away from bread either. Because Eileen worked from 3 to 11, I would be on my own for dinner. Toast is always easy to make. Sometimes I'd have a small pizza delivered. I knew what was happening, but I couldn't seem to stop it. I've got to admit, a lot of my motivation to remain thin was the girls. If I stayed in shape, I could go out with some beautiful women. Now that I was married, the motivation was gone. This wasn't fair to Eileen. She didn't sign up to be married to a man who was 50 pounds overweight. I'm sure she wasn't happy about it, but she wasn't saying anything to me about it. I guess she was going to love me no matter what I looked like.

Chapter 14

The first years of gaining it back

The first 3 years of marriage we spent in an apartment in the same town as my high school. I was hovering around 260 by now. We had remained in the honeymoon stage of our marriage at that time. She couldn't keep her hands off me. But who can blame her? A husband who was now fifty pounds overweight from the time she married me would obviously be a big turn-on to any new bride. We were very happy though, going on our delayed honeymoon to San Diego and San Pedro with a long ride up to wine country. It was a lot of fun. Wine country is a little dangerous. They give you wine in tiny, tiny glasses. It kind of sneaks up on you. After about 25 of those little glasses, you felt little pain. We ended up staying at a bed and breakfast for one night because we were way too drunk to drive back to San Pedro. I don't remember much about the bed and breakfast, but I know the springs on the mattress were squeaky.

As for my career, it took me 3 months to find a job after I graduated. I ended up at Loyola University Medical Center in Pediatric Cardiology. A great Doctor with an unfortunate name (Dr. Ow), yes, I'm serious. He took a chance on a new graduate in a field that was much more difficult than adult Echocardiography. Dr. Ow and a guy named Dr. Husayni taught me so much. I worked there with every child from neonates weighing less than 1 and a half pounds to teenagers with severe congenital heart disease that probably wouldn't live past 30. The only problem with that job was pushing a 600-pound machine around the hospital with hard tires that made it even harder to push. The hospital and clinic wear approximately a mile away from each other. Every couple of days I would have to take that machine down to the basement. A hallway ran all the way from the hospital to the dental school and then to the outpatient center. I usually was always sweating by the time I got to the clinic. Nothing like sweating all over a bunch of babies to make a mother feel confident with you working on their child.

After three years I moved to a level 1 trauma center further south in Oak Lawn, IL. I didn't have a great work experience there from day one, so I won't mention their name hear. I started their pediatric echo lab there and was the only pediatric tech who had past the peds exam at the time. I had become an official registered diagnostic cardiac sonographer. Do you think this hospital would have given me a raise for this achievement? Sorry folks, that's a big fat no. The doctors I moved over there with from Loyola had promised me a specific salary. When I got there, they said the doctors didn't have the right to negotiate for me. So, they lowballed me with an obnoxious salary that was nothing but a lateral move from my old job. I learned a valuable lesson that day. Get everything in writing no matter what. This knowledge became essential when I started my own business. The nice thing was eventually about 10 years after I started my own business, they called me to cover for them because one of their techs had walked out. I charged them so much just to make up for the money I lost that first year I worked there. Sometimes karma is a bitch for businesses too.

I was slowly gaining weight after the first three years of our marriage. I was over 260 when I found out Eileen was pregnant with our first child. She bought me a present for no reason at all. It wasn't my birthday or Christmas; it was just because. When I opened it there was a little pair of baby socks in the box. I had wanted kids since I was one. I loved babies. That's why I chose to work with children. I have to admit this 6'2" 260-pound man cried. I was so happy. Ultrasound was still new for telling whether you were having a boy or a girl. We decided to be surprised.

About three months into the pregnancy, I started to have this unreasonable fear that I was going to die before I saw my child. I had no reason for this fear, I was pretty healthy for an overweight 25-year-old. But the fear was as real as could be. During a dinner date with my beautiful bride, because she craved steak when she was pregnant, we went to a pretty fancy restaurant. In the middle of the meal, I started feeling funny. It started with lightheadedness, followed by dizziness and palpitations. I was sure I was going to faint. I put my head down between my legs, but it didn't seem to help. Then I got this cold sensation running throughout my torso. They almost called an ambulance for me. I refused and just asked Eileen to take me home. The feelings got a little better but were still there by the time I got home. I was sure I had something severe like a brain tumor. After a day of laying on the couch with these feelings coming and going, I finally went to a doctor. They ran a whole bunch of tests. Cat scans, MRIs, EKGs, Echocardiograms, and Carotid ultrasound. Just about every test they could think of. They all came back normal. That's when the doctor told me about panic attacks. He said it was a very intense form of anxiety. He said I may get depressed too because the panic and anxiety can trigger a deeper depression caused by something in my past. I didn't want to believe any of this. At first, I tried to deal with it myself. I started exercising again and tried to take some weight off. The panic attacks continued. I finally went to see a psychiatrist to see if he could help. He gave me some old medication that made me so sleepy I couldn't drive. I was going to lose my job if I didn't find some way of getting better. I tried to find a different psychiatrist and when I finally found one that knew what she was doing, she gave me the reason why this stuff was happening to me and prescribed some medications that helped with the anxiety and panic attacks. Not too long after the anxiety was diagnosed, I started to get depressed. This was as bad as panic and anxiety. I went on meds for that too. It took a while for the depression to get better, but it eventually did. I started to see a psychologist to talk through this problem. It all came back to the way I was raised and my poor body image. He said I needed to accept that it was ok not to look like a GQ model. But that being overweight for all but 4 years of my life and the constant abuse I took from adults like my grandmother down to my classmates.

I was working at Michael Reese Hospital which is now closed. I got in the elevator with a mother and her 3-year-old. When the doors closed the kid pointed up to me and said "Big fat guy" in his three-year-old voice. Several people in the elevator laughed. The mother didn't try to tell him that he shouldn't say things like that. She just accepted that it was ok for her child to make fun of someone like that. I know he was only 3 or 4 but she could have told him that it wasn't nice to make fun of people. Instead, she just smiled and left the elevator with the child in tow. I was madder at the mother than the kid. Why did I take you to this point in my life? These are the kind of things that make you feel inadequate and ugly. I spent a couple of sessions with the psychologist just to get through that little incident. It took me years to realize that all the name-calling and rejection from people because I was overweight, had finally come back to haunt me. I used self-deprecating humor to deal with a lot of the name-calling when I got to be an adult. It was that or beat the shit out of everyone. And we all know how that will go. Spending the night in jail is not what I want to do every time I lose my temper. Plus, beating a 3-year-old up makes me look bad.

When I was at Michael Reese Hospital several of these types of incidents happened. Michael Reese was in a predominantly black neighborhood. The people wear great up there. I never felt out of place. Everyone was happy that you were there to help them. I did echoes on gunshot wounds where the bullet was lodged against the heart. Stab wounds to the heart, and one of the hardest echoes I ever did was a five-year-old child with a bullet in the center of her chest. She survived and did well, but the bullet was resting against her heart. One centimeter more and she would of bleed to death. I hugged my kids that day as soon as I got home from work.

I never felt like I was in danger or anything like that. But I will tell you one thing. Older black women say whatever they want to say. So, if one of them decided I was too fat they would let me know about it. I remember one saying and this is verbatim, "boy, how'd you get so fat?" she had to be 80 years old. I wanted to say, "how'd you get so ugly?" but instead I said, "I like my food, all kinds of food." You have to bite your tongue a lot when you work in the medical field. I always was nice to the patients even if they were assholes. The other thing is elderly people sometimes have this "I'll say whatever I want to say" attitude. I think the elderly shouldn't put up with any kind of shit. But I also think that just because you're old doesn't give you the right to spew vile comments. I know I'm fat. I don't need anyone else in this world to tell me that. I see it every time I get out of the shower. Or I feel it when I try to get up from a chair. You don't have to even mention that I have a weight problem the same way I wouldn't have to mention the large mole on the side of your nose.

Sometimes the biggest source of my anger was the asshole doctors. They were a source of a lot of my psychology sessions. Anger management was something that I had to learn. The large bar I worked in always would call me first if there was a fight because my anger issues were well served as a bouncer. I could take a punch to the jaw and just look back at the guy who threw it and laugh. My pain tolerance is very high. After he hit me, I'd duck low and crack a couple of his ribs. If that didn't stop him, you aim for the nose. That goes for you too, girls. If some guy has his hands on you and you tell him to stop and he doesn't, aim for the nose with a fist (never put your thumb underneath your fingers or you'll break it) or elbow, and then kick him in the nuts and run. Just a little safety tip from an old bouncer that threw a lot of drunk people out of bars. The anger management problem reared its ugly head when I saw a man hit a woman. We would pummel the shit out of him. Every available bouncer would drag him out as quickly and painfully as possible. The problem was sometimes the same girl would get right back into the car with the loser to go home. I would always offer them a cab ride to someplace safe. But some of them you just couldn't get through. Then it was all on them.

Chapter 15

Cause and effect of being overweight

Cause: I can't stop my hand from moving copious food into my mouth.

Effect: Buying all my clothes at the big and tall shops. When you find yourself wearing a 3XLT (three extra-large tall) you know the effect has taken hold.

Yes, It's that simple. You have to get a handle on what you can eat and what you can't. You have to get your brain to trick your stomach into saying "No, I'm not hungry." and tough through it. It sucks. There is no other way to say it. By the way, this is not the section where I become a cheerleader and say "YOU can do it!" You have to be the one who says that. If a trainer helps, go ahead. If getting rid of everything unhealthy in your fridge and cabinets helps you, go ahead. If your cruise control always takes you through McDonald's, buy a new car. Do what you have to do to make it work. Especially if you're a young teenager. Don't miss out on life because you're overweight. Lose it now and enjoy your high school years. Remember, high protein (beef, chicken, even pork) no carbs, no sugars, lots of fruits and vegetables, and enough water to fill a swimming pool.

Chapter 15

Progression

I'd like to say that the weight gain stopped at 260 but I'd be lying. The weight gain continued for so long that it was just a normal part of my life. The weight kept creeping up. Every time I'd have to go to the doctor there would be something new to deal with. The first thing would be the 10-pound weight gain from the last time I was there. The next thing would be something new regarding my health. First, it was high blood pressure. Not so high I was going to have a stroke. But high enough to put me on medicine for it. This was on top of the depression and anxiety medication I was already on. I also wasn't sleeping very well because of a new diagnosis of sleep apnea. I still use a sleep apnea machine every night and take several meds to help me go to sleep. I was still seeing a psychologist every week trying to deal with problems dealing with anxiety and depression. You go back so far into your past that you sometimes see a diaper on yourself. My history was effective in changing the way I looked at the world. I was angry and revengeful. Anyone who slighted me in the least bit became my enemy. I mean that. One bad incident with a doctor at work and they became an enemy. Not just someone I was a little angry at. I'm talking enemy. I'd give them not just a dirty look, but a look that insinuated that if I caught them in the parking garage alone, I would kick their ass. I had arguments with doctors about something I saw on an echocardiogram that they said was an artifact. They would always throw the "I'm the doctor, you're just the tech." Two days later, that so-called "artifact" that I knew was a blood clot caused a massive stroke in the patient. One of these incidents caused the patient to die. If I reported it the doctor's side would always win out because they were evaluated by other doctors. So, I would just highlight the area where the clot was from that point on and washed my hands of it. There were certain doctors I could trust so if something was abnormal, I would point it out to the medical director, and it would usually get taken care of. But the anger toward some of these arrogant docs was severe.

Surprisingly, some of the most argumentative doctors are women. They have this attitude that because there is a history of doctors all being men. The female doctors think they always have something to prove. They love to flex their authoritative muscles at any time they can. Most of the women I worked with I would prefer to see as a patient. But certain ones are so full of themselves that it's hard to take them seriously. I'm not trying to put all doctors, male or female into one basket. I've run into so many arrogant doctors from both sexes that when I finally retired my blood pressure went back down to normal. Most of the time I would recommend seeing a female doctor. Their compassion level is higher than men. It's the nurturing gene (if there is one) that makes most of them great doctors.

My ex-girlfriend the only other woman I fell in love with became a doctor after she had been a physical therapist. I never saw her as a patient (how awkward would that have been) but the reviews she got on google were fantastic. She seemed to be very compassionate and took the appropriate time with each patient to get that review. It's a shame she didn't show me some of that compassion 39 years ago. Ok, I guess I'm still a little mad about that whole situation. But if regress.

My anger management was sometimes curbed by eating. It's hard to stay mad when you're eating a cupcake. Eating your way out of anger was a real thing for me. My father who could unleash his wrath on you and raise your feet off the ground while he was spanking you would follow that punishment by asking me if I wanted a milkshake. If he punished all of us, we all got milkshakes. I think his way of dealing with the guilt of abusing his children was to feed them something delicious. I was furious with my dad for many years after I became an adult because my psychologists said most of my anger was because of the inability to fight back or even argue my point before the discipline was dished out. My mom was responsible for a lot of this too. He would act upon her accusations, and we would get punished without any chance to tell our side of the story. This infuriated me as a child and teenager. The physical discipline wasn't as frequent as we got into our teens, mainly because I was so big. But one time I was in the middle of an argument with my mom and sister because she came in and said I threw rocks against the side of the house. She had just thrown a fist full of rocks at my head. I lashed back by throwing some back at her. My dad and I had just finished painting the house. So, there were these small little chips on the side of the house where the rocks hit. My sister was telling my mom about the rocks, and I was just trying to tell my mom that my sister had thrown rocks at my head first. I even had red marks on my face from the rocks. When I realized, I wasn't going to get a word in edgewise I finally told both of them to shut up so I could tell them what really happened. Unfortunately, my dad had just walked in and heard me tell my mom to shut up. I got punched in the face and then kicked down the stairs. I'm pretty sure he cracked a couple of ribs when he kicked me, and I did hit my head on the way down the stairs. My jaw was so sore I couldn't eat that night. When he finally cooled down, I got in my car (I was 16 when this happened) and disappeared for 12 hours. I came home at 5:00 in the morning. I slept at a friend's house without telling them where I went. When I did come home both parents were at the foot of the stairs extremely angry with me. It was the first time I stood up for myself. I looked at my dad with tears in my eyes and said "the next time you hit me like that I WILL fight back. And you won't like the results." I think I surprised him so much that he didn't know what to say. But my mother always had something to say. She started in on me saying how worried she was when I didn't come home and that she was about to call the police to find me. I said, "why didn't you call the police when your husband hit me in the face and kicked me down the stairs?" I walked right past them and went downstairs to get ready to go work out. I left 15 minutes later with my gym bag and clothes for school. I walked around for a couple of days with a bruise on my jaw and couldn't take in a very deep breath. I didn't talk to either one of them for a week or so. It was very tense around that house for that week. When my dad finally apologized for being so rough with me the damage was already done. From that point on as soon as he would start to yell at me, I'd ball up my fists so he could see me do it. I had to make sure he knew I wasn't ever going to let him beat me again. He never did. This type of abuse most of the time was verbal. Like I said before, my mom had her black belt in guilt. And she wheeled it like an axe. She could cut you down with a sentence.

Now here's where I give my parents an out. Both my parents came from abusive homes. They learned how to parent from their parents. This, unfortunately, is too often the way people learn how to parent. There are so many good resources out there for parenting. If your parents were abusive, IT'S YOUR JOB to break the cycle. When I found out I was going to be a father I knew exactly what not to do. I loved my children to a fault. I probably was too soft on them sometimes. But all four of my children love to talk about what great childhoods they had. My wife is so even-keeled that we were both fair about discipline. We never hit our kids. We also helped them with their homework. I coached basketball, baseball, football, and floor hockey. I was always involved in my boys' sports activities, and I was the kind of coach every parent dreams about. I encourage the best baseball player as much as the worst one. Everyone played. I rotated players in and out no matter if we were winning or losing. Some of the hot-head dads didn't like it but they didn't volunteer to coach. I did. I think my favorite thing to do was put the overweight kid who could play baseball into a shortstop position. No one agreed with what I did, but when the kid made a great play, I was the loudest cheerleader there. I had been a victim of a coach or five that only played the best players in little league. I saw it at the coaching level all the time. And who sat on the bench the most? That's right! The chubby kid. The only sport the overweight kid could play was football. "Stick that fat kid on the offensive line. They won't be able to move him at that weight." That was the thought process in football. I'm from the Chicago area. When the Chicago Bears put refrigerator Perry in the backfield, and he ran over three people to score a touchdown in the Superbowl, you could hear a roar from every overweight person in the world. To see a big guy like that play a position taken by a trim, fat-free, running back was revenge for every offensive or defensive lineman who knew they could play a different position on the football field. Hail to all the offensive and defensive linemen in the world!

Chapter 16

Smoking

When I found out we were going to have our first baby I had been smoking for about 6 years. I had gotten up to two packs a day. I didn't want cigarette smoke around our baby. I needed to quit, and I needed to do it right away. I had tried several times over the years, but I would always go back to them. Finally, after several attempts, I quit. I haven't had a cigarette in 33 years. But there is always a good side and a bad side. The good side was obvious. No more cigarettes meant a healthier Scott and less chance of lung cancer. And also, no smoke around a new baby. But no more cigarettes also meant something had to give. What was it? The give was about another 40 pounds making me an even 300 pounds. I was 25 years old and weighed between 280 and 330 pounds for the next 10 years.

At several points during these 10 years, I was up and down weight-wise. At one time I lost 70 pounds getting me almost to my original weight when I was younger. But it wasn't too long before I started to creep up again. I regained the weight and then some. A couple of years later, I would lose 50 pounds and felt better but still was 250 pounds. Not near my ideal weight but better. I stayed at that weight for a year until the weight kept creeping up again. This is by far the hardest part about being overweight. The ups and downs. How long does this go on? Well, a fricken lifetime. Are there success stories? Hell yes. My brother Keith is a perfect example of someone who was morbidly obese and lost all the weight and has kept it off for 30 years.

Keith is a doctor. A great doctor. Yes, he's my brother and I'm biased but I worked with him during his training. He and I were at his residency hospital. I told him I was going to be there for a while even though I was a private contractor. Keith didn't want to be a cardiologist. He wanted to be an internal medicine doctor. He still took the time to sit with me for an hour or so each day just to learn about my field of pediatric and adult echocardiography. He sat there and listened to me teach him about a test that he would go on to order frequently and wanted to know what the different diagnostic findings were. He's just a great doctor who cares deeply for his patients. I've seen it firsthand.

Now, why do I tell you about Keith? When Keith was an intern, he weighed about 300 pounds. He found himself having to tell patients that it was important to lose weight. I believe one day after telling this to a patient he got a "You shouldn't talk doctor." It hit him hard. He realized that he really shouldn't be telling these patients to lose weight when he was so overweight himself. He knew he had to change his habits so he could be a good example for his patients. Keith is about 6'1" tall. When he got finished losing weight, he was 180. He may have lost even more weight since then because he is thin now. He is an exercise freak and has competed in bicycle races and 10ks often. His biking career ended with a nasty crash causing severe damage to his shoulder and clavicle. He also destroyed a lot of tendons and ligaments. He's still trying to get back to normal, but the damage was so bad he's still afraid to ride.

The fact that Keith had such success makes me feel very proud of him but also very bad about myself. Watching someone you love succeed is always wonderful. But jealous is a nasty wench. I wondered if I was just weaker than my little brother. Something that was hard to swallow. Like I said before, I couldn't be happier for him. He will probably live a lot longer than me.

My ups and downs are my own fault. I have had plenty of time to get out of childhood trauma and bad habits. Now it's me who has all the fault to take. I kept losing and gaining so many times I can't even tell you the honest number of attempts I made. Hovering around 300 became 320, then 340, and then I hit 350 pounds. During this time, I remained active. I put together cribs. Played sports with my boys and finished my basement in two different houses. My weight never stopped me from doing things. Could I do everything? No. But I would surprise a lot of people as to what I could do. I remained at 350 for several years. This has been almost a 30-year process. After losing and gaining during this whole time, I know what it's like to deal with the ebb and flow of weight loss. It took years to find a solution. We'll get into that a little later.

Chapter 17

My brother-in-law

I had a brother-in-law named Jeff. The fact that I have to say "Had" bothers the shit out of me. Jeff went into surgery for a knee replacement at the age of 58. He was in the hospital for 3 days. Being someone who has had multiple knee replacements I know that coming home in 3 days is a testament to Jeff's pain tolerance. Unfortunately, that quick exit from the hospital was a mistake. Along with not sending him home on a blood thinner. My brother-in-law had a massive stroke right in front of his wife. He lingered in the hospital ICU for a couple of days until they put him on the donor list and harvested his organs to save the lives of 6 people. Jeff died at 58 years old.

Jeff and I had a love/hate relationship at least on my end. Jeff was a comedian, the life of any party, and awful hard on me for being overweight. He was pretty relentless with his teasing. Jeff was in perfect shape for a guy of 58. Not an ounce of fat on him. He worked in heating and air conditioning, owning his own business for many years. He was always in hot attics and lifting heavy equipment. He worked his butt off to build a very successful business, and I will always admire him for that.

But his teasing, giving me crap about being fat all the time about being fat hurt. His jabs were minor most of the time. They were little things, like "He can't fit in that booth" or "that seat won't hold him, he's too fat." He never said anything loud enough to attract attention from other tables in a restaurant or at a function of any kind. It was always in close quarters where only my wife's family would hear it. Being insulted in front of strangers is much less painful than insults made around family. It's as painful as being insulted during high school when my friend Rick would insult me in front of girls, I might have a chance of dating. I think back on the time Jeff was alive and the 25 years we spent together as brothers-in-law, and I realize Jeff may have just been trying to be funny. But there is a difference between being funny and using someone else's looks to be funny. I made enough fun of myself for everyone. I didn't need any help. My self-deprecating humor took some of the heat off of me because I took care of the jokes. Leaving no one else the opportunity to make fun of me. But for some reason, Jeff could slip those jokes by and get in a dig at any time.

Everyone in this world has flaws. Some of them are huge, some small. In the big picture of things, I would love to have Jeff alive and making fun of me than what really happened. I would take the teasing back in a heartbeat.

As time went on and I got into my 50's my weight started climbing again. At 360 I had to ask for a table instead of a booth in almost every restaurant. This was also embarrassing. Having some beautiful hostess accidentally bring us to a booth and have to tell her that I wouldn't fit in the booth. Again, my damn fault. But still a form of discrimination. All booths should have a table that can be moved instead of being bolted to the floor. You see, we big people love restaurants. You don't even have to get up to get your food. They bring it right to the table! It's amazing! It's also too easy for us. Not even the simple exercise of getting up to make a meal. With meals being delivered right to you, why would you stay at home to eat?

Getting on a plane also became a problem. At my size fitting into a plane seat was hard to do. And the looks I would get from the people who had to sit in the same row were just short of hateful. My wife is petite, and I hardly ever traveled for business so I could put Eileen in the middle seat and then the person in the third seat would have enough room. I squished Eileen, but she's always cold so a warm body next to her was nice. I tried to give people as much room as they needed but anyone who is over 6 feet tall has trouble fitting in those seats. So being the big and tall version of a human being is not good for us.

Chapter 18

It always catches up to you in some way

In my 50's the bottom started dropping out of my orthopedic health. I always had bad knees from playing sports in high school and college. I had my first knee surgery at the age of 17. By the time I was in my 50's, I had had over 15 knee surgeries. Most of them were scopes, but some of them were the fully open type of surgery. By the age of 56, my weight had gotten up to the highest it had ever been. I weighed 384 pounds. I wanted no part of going under the knife at this weight. It just wasn't safe. I had to lose some weight before I had the knee replacement done. I dealt with the pain and worked out frequently to get my weight down to 325. I felt better about going into surgery. Part of my right knee needed to be replaced.

Unfortunately, that didn't work. I still had pain in the joint. The same doctor decided after a scope to look at the inside of the knee, that a full replacement was necessary. I went into surgery to have the whole knee replacement done wishing we had done this first. When I came out, I had more pain than I had ever had with any other surgery or break in my life. This was pretty brutal. I tend to bleed a lot, so I think I had extra swelling post-op. They take a good portion of bone out of your knee both from the femur and tibia. They also cut the kneecap in half horizontally. They put a cushioning part in the middle of the knee to act as cartilage. After all that work, they bring you back to the room and put you in a machine that moves your knee back and forth to a certain degree marker. Every couple of hours they would move the degree marker up. By the end of the next day, I could bend my knee 90 degrees. After having your knee completely opened, removing the bone needed to place the prosthetic knee in place with both cement and pounding the posts into the femur and tibia, and then placing the fake cartilage (the ortho surgeons call it the hockey puck) they snapped everything into place. There is a reason why I'm explaining this surgery to you. I'll explain later.

Even though I had lost a significant amount of weight before the surgery, I was still 325 pounds. They start you out on a walker and then move you up gradually to crutches. In between, they pretty much torture you in physical therapy. Why, because they really want to. I've worked with these people and they're a sadistic bunch. Just kidding. But not really. It's their job to restore as much range of motion as possible. The further you can bend your knee the better. The doctor is usually pretty happy if they can get you to 120 degrees. I reached

145. I had to work hard to get there because I didn't want to have a limited range of motion. The problem I had was during the rehab of the right knee was my left knee started to fail because it was taking on all that weight. That and years of surgeries and damage, it was bound to fail. When my right knee was finally healed it was time to do the left knee. I wanted the same surgeon, but he was out of the country and couldn't do the procedure. We needed it during a specific week because my wife is a school nurse and also has her doctorate in School Nursing. She teaches in downtown Chicago. Between the two jobs, we had little time she could help me post-op right after the surgery. It amounted to about 2 weeks. The doctor who filled in said he worked with my doctor often and would be able to do the surgery without a problem. He replaced the knee, and I went through rehab all over again. One day approximately 6 months later I was walking out to the mailbox when I heard a pop in my left knee and then felt my knee crack. Not a lot of significant pain, but I knew something wasn't right when I came in and was able to pull my tibia (lower leg bone) forward and back. It would crack every time this happen which was often. I called the doctor and ended up there the same day. He said the knee had come apart and would have to be replaced again. On the way home I was in tears knowing I would have to go through the whole thing again. And this was going to be a different kind of surgery called a revision surgery. It's a surgery that is for someone who has already had a replacement. They put in deeper posts and still have to trim the bone more. I know what you're saying. He's got to be done now. What else could go wrong? And you only have two knees. That's what I said. Unfortunately, because I couldn't exercise, my weight shot up to 350 again. I was still able to walk after the 3rd replacement, but a little slower and with a cane. Then just for kicks, my right knee started to give me pain on the lateral side (outside) of the knee. When they took an x-ray of it there was a very large bone spur growing off the remnant of my kneecap. It was rubbing against the bone and the prosthesis, so it had to be removed. Simple

surgery, right? Just go in there and grind the spur off with a scope. Well, it didn't happen that way. The bone spur was much larger and thicker than they thought it would be, so they had to open up the knee along the top and chisel off the bone spur. They were successful and got all of it off. This surgery didn't require a lot of physical therapy, so I wasn't that worried about the recovery time. Everything should be easy, right? Wrong. Three or four days after the surgery I started to have swelling and significant pain. When I got up from the couch and let out a yell, my wife told me if I didn't call the doctor, she was going to hit me with a frying pan. I didn't want that because she's got a mean right hook. I could barely move or bend my right knee because of the swelling. When I called the doctor, they wanted to see me immediately. Unfortunately, the doc was located in Chicago which meant a bumpy ride down to the hospital. If you've ever had the pleasure of driving in Chicago during pothole season, you know how bumpy it can get. I got there and watched them take the dressing off. The bottom two stitches were open and the stuff oozing out of my knee didn't smell very nice. They aspirated the knee (sticking a long needle in the knee and removing the extra fluid from the knee) the color of the fluid wasn't pretty and they were able to remove 100cc's. That's a lot of fluid. He said he was going to put me on a high-dose oral antibiotic and sent me home. 3 days later, I was back, this time chasing the doctor to another hospital to have the knee washed out in surgery hoping that would be enough to get rid of the infection. This procedure happened three times. Finally, because nothing was getting better, they put a pick line in (a large port to hook up an IV every day) and then went in and replaced the knee again. I had to endure IV vancomycin twice a day for 7 weeks. The port had to be flushed every two days so that was another thing they were watching. All this happened because some physician's assistant was in too big a hurry to sew up my wound properly. After 8 weeks of dealing with the infection, I started the rehab process again. 8 more weeks of that and I was finally done. Technically, I had 5 knee replacements on two knees. Why do I bring you through this sad sack story? Because if I had been at a normal weight all my life there would have been a good chance that I wouldn't have ever had to have a knee replacement at all. Or at least not till I was in my seventies.

Let's add one more thing to the picture that eventually landed me on disability. I've also had back problems since I started lifting heavy patients in physical therapy. (I'll blame Kathy for this because I followed her around like a puppy dog. And heaven forbid she should have to lift anyone on her own. I would do anything for her) I spent time in the hospital when I was 21 for a severe back strain. That was the beginning. Now add 50 pounds 4 years later and you have a very large stomach pulling your back forward and putting a lot of pressure on the disks in your back. When I was at my heaviest, I was putting an extra 175 pounds on my back. I developed a couple of bad disks. I had many epidural injections. They were Mickey Mouse bandages on a gunshot wound. My back was a mess. The biggest problem was called spinal stenosis. It's arthritis in the spinal canal. It eventually puts severe pressure on the spinal cord and causes severe spasms in the back and down the leg. I couldn't take it anymore. I had to have a 3-level laminectomy. A laminectomy is a surgery where they remove bone in the spine to relieve the pressure on the spinal cord. Some of the vertebrae had to be altered, so the pressure could be removed from the spinal cord. After that, my surgeon told me my back would not be able to tolerate pushing the echo machine around the hospital. The new machines weigh between 300 to 400 pounds. My back would not hold up to pushing that machine anymore. Now, I've been on disability for 4 years, and a good reason that has occurred is that I've had a significant obesity problem for most of my life. They say you eventually pay for your bad habits. This was my first payment. I was and still am an orthopedic nightmare.

Chapter 19

Limitations of movement

The aftermath of this disaster I call the "missing years" because I was under anesthesia so much, I was unconscious more than conscious. But in all seriousness, what all of the crap I went through really meant was a limitation of movement. My ability to exercise effectively was long gone. Treadmills and ellipticals hurt. I thought a recumbent bike might be better. I was wrong. The only thing I can do is take a walk outside at a slow to medium pace. Is it something? Yes. Is it enough? No. Was I a big cardio person before all the orthopedic problems? No. I can still lift weights with my upper body and can do some lightweight work with my legs. But I lose interest fast in the workout world. It bores me. It always has. Even when I was 19 and used it as my main exercise to lose weight. I can't seem to gather any interest in it anymore. It's harder to build muscle mass at 61. So, you have to work twice as hard and twice as long to get the same muscle mass as I did when I was 19. The need to exercise to lose weight is debatable now. Some experts say that you can lose weight by eating a high protein, low carbohydrate, low sugar diet. Is this easy to do? Hell no. It takes incredible discipline. Discipline is very hard to sustain long term. Every January 1st of every year millions of people make the resolution to lose weight. Most succeed in the first or second week. Then someone has a birthday and there is chocolate cake. Suddenly you think "one piece won't hurt." Then that turns into "well, I already had 1 piece of cake, one more won't hurt." Now the sugar is in your body. So, the next time you have something with sugar in it put in front of you, you'll break. Then before you know it, losing weight is no longer a priority. Then it's over. Maybe you'll try again this year, maybe not. You may find yourself on the next January 1st making the same resolution. You may need to lose 10 pounds or 100 pounds. Both goals can be achieved by an extremely strong person who has the determination or the true need to lose weight. What do I mean by that? You need to lose weight after a heart attack. You need to lose weight when you find out you have type ll diabetes. You need to lose weight when you find out that your organs are starting to show the age of a 75-year-old. You need to lose weight when your wife or husband doesn't want to make love to you anymore because of your weight. The last one would hurt more than all the others combined. It doesn't say very much about your spouse, because if better or worse was said by both of you, consider this part to be the worst. You could be supportive and try to help your husband or wife eat right. But you have to do it gently. If you think yelling at someone you supposedly love is going to work, you might as well pack your bags now and find some skinny person who will never love you as much as your husband or wife did. I have the most wonderful wife. She has been beside me through all of these problems, including being married to a fat guy. That's what she has probably heard a time or two from some of her friends or family members. Yet she's still here, and she still loves me. Because being overweight comes with the problem of having no self-confidence, I always worry. Worry that she'll break someday and find some skinny guy and leave me in the dust. We've been together for 39 years, so I think I'm safe. She has always been there. When I think back to that time, I left her after the first month of our dating for a woman who had no idea what she wanted other than to find a guy to cheat on her fiancé with. Maybe it was deeper than that, I'll never know now that she's passed. But when Eileen let me back into her life, I grabbed onto her, and I'll never let go.

I want to change subjects now and tell you about my hatred of mirrors. When you are up there in weight, not 10 pounds, I'm talking 50 to 100 pounds. A mirror is not your friend. Especially a full-length mirror. And God forbid you to walk by one naked. The puke factor moves up to 10 quickly. It's been my enemy for so long that it's going to be on the same level as the 100-year war. But the absolute worst place to find yourself is in a tuxedo shop when they put you in front of that full-length triple-sided mirror. The horror! The only thing I could think of that could be worse is if I were naked in front of those mirrors. Or maybe a nudist colony filled with swimsuit models.

I also have a real problem looking at pictures of myself. Even the ones with my grandchildren. That sounds awful, I know. It's just looking at those beautiful children sitting with me and me dwarfing them because I'm so big makes me crazy. I know it shouldn't matter. All the kids care about is the fact that they're with papa. And I know it, but it still makes me so self-conscious. I have pictures of me when I was thin. My wedding picture is on canvas right on my dresser in my bedroom. I don't mind looking at that one. It was the last time I had a good self-image of myself. The last couple of chapters will explain how I've come to terms with my self-image problems. Although a person who has had such a poor self-image for as many years as I have will never be perfect or completely accepted. It's just the nature of the beast. Funny, that was one of my favorite albums when I was young. Nature of the Beast by April Wine.

Chapter 20

The health problems

This is the scary part of my story. The overall health problems. The ones that go along with being both older and overweight. The one that has been with me for the longest is High blood pressure. It is often the first thing that affects an overweight person. Because of my background in cardiology, I want to try to explain what high blood pressure does to the body.

There are two components to high blood pressure (which is also called hypertension) The systolic blood pressure is the upper number. The diastolic blood pressure is the lower number. The upper number is the pressure in the artery when the heart pumps blood into the arteries. The diastolic blood pressure is the time when the heart rests and the pressure in the arteries is lower. So, 120/80 is normal blood pressure but so is 112/72, and 132/84 are all good pressures. When it gets up over 140/90 then you have mild hypertension. As it rises to pressures like 180/110 you may have a stroke or a heart attack. I've seen blood pressure as high as 240/140. That's a critical situation. Go to the Emergency Room, now! You could have a stroke within minutes. You need to be on medication to bring the pressure down. If you don't take your medicine the heart will get enlarged. It can either get thicker or dilate. Both are serious problems. Both can cause congestive heart failure. That goes along with shortness of breath. You can end up on oxygen for the rest of your shortened life. Obviously, these are worst-case scenarios. But it was the earliest problem I faced. This is extremely common in overweight people. I pulled something off the Mayo Clinic website. It even floored me. Here's the quote: "Fat is not an inert substance. It is a very active substance that puts out a lot of chemicals that damage our arteries," says Dr. Kopecky. "Fat damages our body tissues. It actually makes our bodies less sensitive to insulin so we're more prone to being a diabetic."

And extra fat makes your circulatory system work overtime.

"Every pound of weight we put on is 5 miles of blood vessels. If your heart beats 100,000 times a day, that's 500,000 miles a day for one pound of fat," says Dr. Kopecky.

That's also the reason that people who are overweight have an increased heart rate. Normal sinus rhythm produces a heart rate of 60 to 100 beats per minute. That's at rest. Put your index and middle fingers on the right side of your neck right between the center and the side of the neck. Push down a little and you should feel your heart rate. You may have to move around a little until you find it. Once you feel your pulse look at your phone or watch. Set a timer on your phone for 1 minute. Find your pulse in your neck first. Then start the timer and start counting your pulse rate. When you get to one minute that is your heart rate. See if it's high. You may have a normal heart rate, or you may have an increased heart rate if you are significantly overweight. If you're reading this and you just happen to be in good shape, your resting heart rate may be low. Maybe in the '50s. People who run marathons or consistently run 10k races can have a rate in the 40s. I saw a triathlete who had a sleeping heart rate of 32. If this happened to a normal person, they would have to go to the cath lab to have a pacemaker put in.

So, these two things are important to monitor when you are overweight. High blood pressure can cause so many problems both short and long-term. Mainly long-term but its damages are hard to reverse. A high heart rate means your heart works harder every minute than it needs to. My resting heart rate at my heaviest was around 120 beats per minute. That's not good at all. I had to go on a blood pressure medicine that also had what's called a beta blocker in it to slow my heart rate. The beta blocker is mainly for blood pressure but also has a pulse rate effect. Beta-blockers are an old drug, but still very effective. If your pulse rate is high, your doctor may put you on this medication.

The last thing I want to say on this subject is PLEASE go see a doctor once a year. New drugs to help with weight loss come out all the time. Also, there are surgical procedures (which I will get into later) that are specifically designed for the morbidly obese or even the obese. These procedures produce results almost immediately if you stick with the program.

One of the other problems that are very prominent in morbidly obese people is sleep apnea. It can be a problem with all kinds of increased weight gain. What happens is you start to snore loudly because of the extra weight that gathers on the front of your neck. I was able to find a good explanation of sleep apnea at the Mayo clinic site. Here it is: Sleep apnea[3] is a potentially serious sleep disorder in which breathing repeatedly stops and starts. You may have sleep apnea if you snore loudly or feel tired even after a full night's sleep.

The main types of sleep apnea are:

- **Obstructive sleep apnea,** the more common form that occurs when throat muscles relax.

---

3. http://www.mayoclinic.org/diseases-conditions/sleep-apnea/basics/definition/con-20020286

- **Central sleep apnea,** which occurs when your brain doesn't send proper signals to the muscles that control breathing.
- **Complex sleep apnea syndrome,** also known as treatment-emergent central sleep apnea, occurs when someone has both obstructive sleep apnea and central sleep apnea.

The signs and symptoms of obstructive and central sleep apnea overlap, sometimes making the type of sleep apnea more difficult to determine. The most common signs and symptoms of obstructive and central sleep apneas include:

- Loud snoring, which is usually more prominent in obstructive sleep apnea
- Episodes of breathing cessation during sleep witnessed by another person
- Abrupt awakenings accompanied by shortness of breath, which more likely indicates central sleep apnea
- Awakening with a dry mouth or sore throat
- Morning headache
- Difficulty staying asleep (insomnia)
- Excessive daytime sleepiness (hypersomnia)
- Attention problems
- Irritability

Consult a medical professional if you experience, or if your partner notices, the following:

- Snoring loud enough to disturb the sleep of others or yourself
- Shortness of breath, gasping for air, or choking that awakens you from sleep
- Intermittent pauses in your breathing during sleep
- Excessive daytime drowsiness, which may cause you to fall asleep while you're working, watching television, or even

driving

Many people don't think of snoring as a sign of something potentially serious, and not everyone who has sleep apnea snores. But be sure to talk to your doctor if you experience loud snoring, especially snoring that's punctuated by periods of silence.

Ask your doctor about any sleep problem that leaves you chronically fatigued, sleepy, and irritable. Excessive daytime drowsiness (hypersomnia) may be due to sleep apnea or to other disorders, such as narcolepsy. Treatment can ease your symptoms and may help prevent heart problems and other complications.

As complex as that sounds, when you take it in little bites, it's not so hard to understand. One of the things it didn't mention is one of the long-term possibilities of sleep apnea is pulmonary hypertension. This is a disease of the lungs where the pressure on the right side of the heart goes up high and ends up enlarging the right side of the heart. The valve (tricuspid) becomes insufficient, and between the leaky valve and the increased pressure the right heart may begin to fail. Right-sided congestive heart failure is as serious as left-heart congestive heart failure. I guess I should have explained the right and left-sided heart sections. The left heart is for pumping blood to the body. The right heart only pumps blood to the lungs. So, it's like you have two hearts that pump blood to different areas of the body. The heart is one big loop. Oxygen-poor blood enters the right heart from the two big veins that bring blood back to the right side of the heart. The blood is pumped through the right heart to the lungs where the blood is oxygenated and then brought to the left side of the heart via the pulmonary veins. The left side then pumps the oxygenated blood throughout the body and then the whole process starts over again with the next heartbeat. It's nothing but a big circle of blood flow.

The newest problem

So, I am trying to be a writer now. I've written some romance novels (don't judge me, I like romance novels) I've also have written a couple of paranormal-type novels. I like to sit in my recliner to write because I'm more comfortable and the pain in my knees and back are less reclined. But a problem arose just recently. When I sit for a time writing, as I go from a sitting to a standing position, my blood pressure drops. Sometimes I go from a normal sitting blood pressure of 122/76 to a pressure of 70/30. It really should make me pass out. I do get very lightheaded and sometimes feel like I'm going to faint. I have to find a chair rather quickly. Once I sit for a little while, I'm fine. This is called orthostatic hypotension. Hypo means low in this word; tension means pressure. So, in the middle of standing up, my blood pressure drops significantly. Enough to make me faint and then fall. A fall at my size would be extremely dangerous. Also, the older you get the more susceptible you are to brain bleeds if you hit your head, you can die just from that. A fainting spell for a guy that weighs 270 pounds can cause the head injury we talked about, a broken hip, and other broken bones too.

Chapter 21

The biggest decision of my overweight life

I had gotten back up to 380 pounds a couple of years ago. So, at 59, I made a decision that changed my life for the better. I went into a bariatric care center and listened to an introduction seminar about the gastric sleeve operation. This is something I was against for so long. I didn't want anybody changing the way food was processed in my body. Was so fed up with being morbidly obese that this was now my only option. I had lost a significant amount of weight on my own many times during my adult life. But now that I couldn't really exercise efficiently, I needed help. After researching and watching many operations on healthcare sites that did the procedure. Even YouTube had videos of the surgery.

This is an explanation of the gastric sleeve operation that I had from the University of Chicago Medical Center: During a verticle gastric sleeve procedure, the stomach is permanently reduced to about

15 percent of its original size, leaving a sleeve-shaped portion that can hold less food and is resistant to stretching.

So basically, they remove a large portion of your stomach and then strengthen that part of the new stomach, so it doesn't stretch. So, here are the only things you really need to know. This is surgery. And surgery on a significantly obese person is dangerous. There can be complications. Any good bariatric surgeon has a team of people who know the special needs of a morbidly obese patient. The anesthesiologist will have been trained to use only the minimum of anesthesia to lessen the effects of the drugs used to put you to sleep. The procedure is done with a scope that allows all of the work to be done with minimal surgical recovery. I only had 5 small holes from the surgery. The only one that is bigger is the incision they used to remove the section of the stomach that they had to remove. After they remove the extra part of the stomach they sew up the remaining stomach. They stitch up all the incisions and pull your big butt onto a bed and take you to recovery. Don't worry, they do it gently.

I spent 1 night in the hospital to make sure there are no complications. I was sent home in a little bit of pain, but it wasn't that bad. You're on clear liquids for a while (maybe 3 days). After that, more of a full liquid diet. Like cream of chicken soup and other things. Then the protein starts. I don't remember what follows that, but I can tell you, the amount of food you can eat has been cut into about ⅓ or less of the food you use to be able to eat. Because your stomach is so small, you fill up so fast that you're almost guaranteed to lose weight. All you have to do is follow the high protein low carb diet that they give you. They like you to exercise if you can after your incisions are healed. You use your abdominal muscles a lot more than you think. They don't want you to do too much. Walking, some light weights, things like that. I could not believe how quickly I filled up when I ate. My eyes were used to putting these large portions on my plate. I would have to throw away all the food that was left on my plate. My wife had to start fixing my plate like I was a 2-year-old because I had no idea how to put the proper portion on my plate. When she did fill my plate, it always looked like the smallest amount of food. But sure enough, it would be the exact amount of food that would fill me up.

The weight started dropping off of me at an alarming rate. If I remember right, I lost 25 pounds in the first couple of weeks or so. It just changes your whole outlook on everything. Suddenly, you want to eat healthier to help you drop even more weight. After the first month, I lost 25 pounds. It kept going at that rate. My clothes started becoming loose. After the 2nd month, I was down about 40 pounds. I went from a 3xlt shirt to a 2xlt. I had to buy some new jeans. I also had to punch some more holes into my belt. This was always fun to do. I have a leather punch on my Swiss army knife. Every time I would open it I felt better. After a couple more weeks I was down 50 pounds. People were starting to notice. Family especially. My sister-in-law said, "I can get my arms all the way around you!" That meant a lot so thank you, Jean. Things don't always progress that fast, but I always lost some weight. After a couple more months I had lost enough weight to buy extra-large shirts. I hadn't been in an extra-large shirt since the original time I lost weight when I was 18. This was monumental for me. I had lost 70 pounds by then and everyone was noticing. Friends couldn't believe what I looked like. They dropped every compliment they could on me and it felt wonderful. 8 months after the surgery, I hit the 100-pound mark. That was the first goal. I took a picture of the scale and sent it to all my kids. 284 pounds. I felt so much better. All my orthopedic problems were better. Especially my back. I used to have an epidural shot near the L5 vertebrae every 3 months. I haven't had one in nearly a year. I'd like to say my knees are much better but that would be a lie. My knees are still bad. But they were such a mess before the surgery I'm not surprised there not better.

Things slowed down from there. I lost another 20 pounds but then gained 15 back. I was eating these peanut butter granola bars that I thought would be a good snack. They have as many calories in them as some candy bars. If I stopped eating those peanut butter bars, I could reach my final goal of 250 pounds. I would be ok with that. I'm a big guy with a barrel chest and large shoulders. So, if I get down to 250 I'll be pretty happy. Anything after that is gravy. I guess I shouldn't say gravy to people who are trying to lose weight.

The smaller stomach is still there, and I know that because I just ordered spaghetti at a fancy Italian restaurant last night. I ate 2 small meatballs and two forkfuls of spaghetti and that was it. I took home a carry-out container filled with spaghetti and some leftover meatballs. You just can't eat that much. I get pain in the abdomen if I eat too much. You feel the fullness hit you and you know if you have one more bite you're going to be in pain. It's the best warning signal you get when it comes to overeating. Because this surgery can be overridden by overeating and stretching the stomach. My son is a nurse in an emergency room. He had a guy present at the hospital with severe abdominal pain. He told the ER staff that he was coming home after having the gastric sleeve surgery and was so hungry from not eating anything but clear liquids. He decided to stop at Burger King and order 2 whoppers. He ate both of them stretching the newly formed stomach so much it tore. He started bleeding severely and passed away on the operating room table. So, if you don't follow the rules, bad things can happen. I don't know how this guy did it. The pain must have been incredible and yet he kept eating. It also had to travel up his esophagus to some degree. That much food in a stomach that is the size of a banana doesn't seem possible. But if he just kept stuffing food in the new stomach would dilate enough to burst. The pain must have been incredible. You have to follow the rules in this surgical journey. I did follow the rules and had success. I still have a way to go, but I'll get there. If you see a new 61-year-old male swimsuit model hit the scene, you'll know it's me.

Chapter 22

So, let's finish this up

I want this section to be for adolescents and teenage kids.

I want to tell you something. If you don't lose the weight now you will suffer through your grade school and high school years. You will be teased. You will be made fun of for just being you. It won't matter how good of a person you are inside, which is a damn shame because you will be ignored by the opposite sex or the same sex. Whatever your preference. You may be picked last every time a pick-up game in some sport starts. If you're a girl, you may not be invited to go with the other girls to the mall or for a sleepover. It's time to get help. Here is the help. Talk to your parents. You need their help. Obesity runs in the family. If your parents are big, the chances of you being fat are high. You have to get them to buy you healthy foods. Maybe you can get your parents to start eating healthily too. It's easier to have people do this with you. You can make it a little contest. You don't have to lose a lot per week. Maybe 2 pounds or so a week. But you have to stick with it. Have some fruit for breakfast and some sort of protein for lunch. Dinner can be chicken, meatloaf, steak, hamburger, or cheeseburger without a bun. Lots of vegetables. Popcorn without a lot of butter for a snack before you go to bed while you're watching a movie. Remember, high in protein, low in carbohydrates, and low in sugar. This doesn't sound like fun, does it? Well, let me tell you it will be a lot easier to do than it will be to tolerate the teasing and ridicule that will occur on almost a daily basis. DON'T LET THIS HAPPEN! I don't care if it takes you a year. It will be so worth it. Don't forget to walk every day. It can be on a treadmill or just taking a walk outside. Buy some arm weights to use. Small to start with. Maybe 5 pounds each. Do arm curls. Lay on your back and push the weights up above your chest. Sit-ups are great too. Start out slow. Maybe do 10 or 20 to start with. Then work your way up. Try maybe 5 more each day. Even one more per day is great. The most important thing is screen time. Screen time in front of a video game, an iPad, or even a plain old tv has to be limited. Set a timer on your phone or just look at a clock. Play whatever game you want to play for one hour. Then walk away! It's time to go outside. Ride a bike to your friend's house. Do some work around the house to help your mom and dad out. Anything physical. And keep going until dinner time. This is assuming this is a school day. If you had gym class today and did something physical like playing basketball or soccer, then you can skip the exercise that day. But if you stood in right field and waited around for a baseball to come to you that's not physical. You need to move. The more you move, the quicker the weight will come off. Stay on the diet! There are some treats you can have. I used to have cut-up strawberries and cool whip. Is that the perfect snack, no. But it's not processed as much as a Little Debbie Snack. Learning how to enjoy fruits and vegetables is an important part of this weight loss journey. Adding sliced almonds and garlic to green beans is very tasty. You can spice up lots of vegetable dishes.

If you don't move this won't work for you! I don't think they do gastric sleeve operations on children or early teens unless the obesity is so severe the child or teen may die if they don't lose weight. Hopefully, you've read this entire book. It's important to finish it. But for you adolescents and teens, this is your chance to change your life. Not a little. A lot! Want to have a girlfriend or a boyfriend? Start today so all that will happen naturally. Start today so you can go to the homecoming and prom dance. Start today so you'll be invited to parties and over to friends' houses. Although, if you have to be thin to be invited to your friend's house then he or she is not really a friend. This statement is for the boys: Someday, you will see a girl in high school that will make you think that there is no way any other girl is as pretty and nice as her. If you are thin and in good shape, you'll have the confidence to talk to her and eventually, ask her out. Even if it's only to a football game or a walk around the mall. Trust me, when that day comes, you'll look back and say, "I'm so glad I lost all that weight when I did."

Now for you girls: This will be hard. But remember, no matter how hard you try you won't be able to cover up an extra 40 pounds. You have to focus on what's important. Your ability to lose weight will make all the difference in the world. Remember too, that boys are much less mature than girls. They will have no problem making fun of you for being fat. And that's just how it is. Boys are mean. They won't care that you are funny and sweet and a wonderful person who is full of love. I am ashamed to be a man sometimes. Especially during my teenage years. Even though I was overweight, I would never look at a girl that was heavy and think "I should go out with her." Even though I did go out with a couple of girls who had an extra 10 or 20 pounds on them. I wasn't special for doing this. I liked these girls because they were funny and pretty. But I never looked at a girl as a possible girlfriend who was significantly overweight. And that's all on me. I was just as much of a shit as any other teenage boy, and I was 90 pounds overweight! Talk about hypocrisy.

The instructions for the girls are no different than they are for the boys. You have to exercise. Like I said before, take a walk. Or join a class at the gym. There are so many classes available for women at most gyms that you can exercise every day and eat right the weight will come off if you stick with it. Then you have to adopt that healthy lifestyle for the rest of your life. Does that mean you can never have a piece of cake from the Cheesecake Factory? Hell no! But you can't have a piece every week. There is no reason you can't have a little treat once in a while. It's the overloading of carbs and sugar on an everyday basis. You can't keep eating the way you are now and expect the weight to fall off. You can't keep sedentary and think the weight is going to fall off. This is hard! But this will be so worth it. Watching the weight come off is so exciting. Even if you can only drop a couple of pounds a week. Remember too, that the more exercising you do the faster the weight will come off. Don't feel self-conscious about exercising. If someone is looking at you because you're big, ignore them. Just do your class at the gym and move on. Someday, that woman will not believe how much weight you've lost. That's if she is as committed to exercising. A lot of people start an exercise program only to give up in a month when it gets hard to make time for it. Because they want to watch Netflix and binge on some show they've already seen twice. When they do that, you'll be at the class exercising.

One other thing I would like to recommend to everyone reading this right now. Do not weigh yourself every day! Weigh yourself once a week at the same time on the same day. Do it in the morning before you get in the shower. Don't have your coffee or a bottle of water first! Take all your clothes off and just get up and get on the scale. As for scales get a good one. Some digital scales can weigh a person all the weigh up to over 450 pounds. I like digital scales because you get a more accurate reading. Slowly get on the scale. Don't step on it like you're running up a flight of stairs. Sometimes I would put the scale in a doorway and hold both sides of it when I step up on the scale. The weight will still be accurate.

The last thing I have to say to this group of adolescents and teens is don't subject yourself to the cold-hearted abuse that I had to put up with when I was your age. Remember, I suffered long-term damage from this abuse. Damage that made at least 2 members of the psychology world much richer. Obviously, it wasn't all because of this specific problem of being overweight. Just remember that you can avoid all the pain I suffered by just changing your life path. You can be the thin kid instead of a fat kid. You'll be happier, healthier, and ready for the steps you'll take to adulthood. You will live happier. Not because your thin, but because your life will be easier in so many ways. Your health will be better, you'll have your choice of boys that like you, and knowing boys there will be a lot of them.

Don't wait to start. One of the biggest mistakes I used to make is delaying the start of changing my life. I would say "I'll start my diet on Monday" and then pig out for however many days were left till Monday." This thought process just delays the start and adds extra pounds that you now have to deal with because you ate like a pig from Wednesday till Sunday night when you had a hot fudge sundae before you went to bed. Now you have an extra 2 or 3 pounds to lose before you get to the weight you were at in the beginning. I hate the word diet. The word die is in it and that can't be good. As soon as you read all the rules for the diet you want to die. That's why I found the simplest diet I could find that made the most sense. When I read about The Atkins Diet, I liked how it explained the evils of carbohydrates. And how high protein helped build muscles and also fill you up. The rest of it talked about how important it was to drink a lot of water too. It would keep you feeling full. I never peed so much in my life.

Now you may find a diet that fits your needs better. Please stay away from fad diets. Eating nothing but grapefruit is just wrong. How long can you go on just grapefruit? Not long. Then you'll be right back to the poor diet you started with two weeks ago. And now you hate grapefruit too. I was not a fan of counting calories either. I'm not that ambitious. And add cards to the situation that you put away after you eat a certain number of calories. It's just too much work. I just like simple. High protein / low carbohydrates and low sugar way of life work the best for weight loss. It also works faster if you have a lot of weight to lose. As time goes on, you can add foods that you like. Maybe a small potato with some butter on it. Or the occasional treat like a small piece of cake. You'll be vibrating after that because of all the sugar. Once you've been off sugar for a long time your body will react to a sugar influx. Exercise in some way. Even if it's in a chair. People who are 600 pounds and have gastric sleeve surgery start exercising in bed by doing simple arm lifts. It doesn't seem like it would make a big difference but we're talking about a person who barely moves all day. Walking may be so limited due to shortness of breath or just the fact that their legs we're not strong enough to support them. If these people remain dedicated, they drop weight very fast. Eventually, they can go for a walk to exercise. It may be only in the house but they're moving and that's all that matters. I know that these people are going to die if they don't change things. I feel sorry for these people because even if they lose let's say more than half of their excess weight there will be many surgeries to remove excess skin from the weight loss. If the skin is breaking down because of infection or fungus insurance should cover it. If they're doing it just to look better the cost is on them. Plastic surgeons are not cheap. And the removal of a large amount of skin is a dangerous surgery. There can be a lot of bleeding during the surgery. It's a long road back for those people. It can be done, though. Men also have to have some surgery too. Mainly the stomach area, but it's less than most women usually have to have. Not everyone chooses to have surgery to reduce the extra skin. If you wait long enough, the skin does stretch back into its originally tight form. But it can take years. This is where the gym may help. Improving muscle tone will help with skin tightening. But it's a lot of work, so be ready to be there 6 days a week.

Chapter 23

What could have happened

That's the big question. How much longer do you intend to put up with this rollercoaster of pain? Being overweight hurts. Physically and mentally. But mainly for you teenagers out there. You can stop all this pain by stopping the weight gain early. Before all the rejection and nasty comments. Before the teasing, and the loss of friends just because you are overweight. You see, these shallow people will not let you into their circles just because you have a different body shape than them. These people are not your friends. They may have once been, but not anymore. You will retain real friends. The ones who are really your friends. They won't care that you are overweight. They will defend you when other people make fun of you. They will also include you in whatever they are doing. Going to parties, sitting at a good table at lunch, and even trying to set you up with the opposite sex. Friends come in and out of your life like busboys in a restaurant. They may be there for years. They may only be their high school and then disappear into a job and family. Don't worry, you'll see them at the reunion.

Don't let the pain get to you. It will slow you down. I endured years of pain before I realized that I could change things. I missed so many milestones in high school. All because I waited. I ate whatever I wanted to and let myself get to the point where I couldn't find a way out. It's like being trapped on a figure 8 racetrack. You go around on a track and hope you don't run into something or someone. The first one that may be hitting your car may represent a nasty comment by the girl you liked in junior high school. Your car is dented, but you go on anyway. 4 or 5 laps later someone says, "what did that fat ass do this time?" If you remember, my grandma said that. You take another hit to your car. It's damaged a little more, but you keep going because you're a glutton for punishment. You know you should pull off that track and re-train your car to avoid accidents. Now substitute your car for your body and repair all the dents. The nasty remarks, the being picked last in gym class because of your weight. Not being able to get a date for any of the dances. Always being the third wheel. Get off the track and repair yourself. Train yourself to eat right and exercise. Even if it takes a year, the next time you get on the track, no one will be able to hit you because you'll be just like everyone else. You'll be at a normal weight.

Remember those jerks who made fun of you? I hope you run into one of them after you lose all the weight. This was the best feeling for me after I lost weight. Running into a person who had written you off as a possible friend or date is the best feeling. Especially if the girl doesn't recognize you. Someone I liked in high school. A girl with long brown hair and beautiful blue eyes. She was always nice to me but made it clear that I was to be relinquished to the friend zone. I was sent to the friend zone so many times in high school I could teach the rules of being in the friend zone. Years later I was in a restaurant with Eileen and L.G. was in the restaurant with a bunch of her friends from work. Someone was retiring so I didn't want to make a scene of the whole thing. I excused myself from the table telling Eileen I was about to get some revenge. She didn't mind at all. I got up and went to L.G. who was sitting near the end of the table. She saw me coming and smiled at me. I thought she recognized me but when I got up to the table with her still smiling and interested, I said to her "did you go to Tinley Park High School? She said she did. I said "You graduated in 1980, right? She nodded her head. She said, "do I know you?" I replied "do you remember this fat guy who use to follow you around all the time. She said she didn't." that kind of hurt but she still hadn't recognized me. My hair was long, and it had been permed to go along with the rock star look. I also had a full beard. I finally said "I guess I let you off the hook because you still don't know who I am." she said "It's killing me! Please tell me. I looked her in the eyes and said "Scott Moss." She lost it practically tackling me to the ground when she found out. She said "Oh My God how much weight did you lose? I said 90 pounds. She then said the one thing I wanted to hear. She said, "We should go out sometime to catch up." I said, "I think I would have a hard time getting that passed my wife." I pointed at Eileen who waved at her. L.G. reluctantly waved back. Nothing feels better when they can't figure out who you are. Give them your name and watch them react. Not only is it fun, but there is also a level of revenge included in these meetings. There's a movie out from probably 10 years ago called "Best Friends" with Ryan Reynolds. This movie is almost like an autobiography of my life. Except I never got the high school girl. I did get her to watch the movie and told her that the story was about her and me. After she watched it she called me and her voice was breaking. She said she just watched the movie and never had an idea that I felt that way about her. I said "how can you tell me that? I did everything to protect you. And when Rick broke your heart I took a night off of work to take you to see Elton John without even knowing if you'd go with me. After I bought the tickets, you called Rick and said something had come up and you couldn't go out to talk with him that night. It was such a win for me. We had nosebleed seats, but we danced to his music and had lots of fun. You even let me dance with you during the song "Your Song" and I sang the whole song in your ear when you had your head on my shoulder. I'm positive she won't remember any of that. But someone as sentimental as me will always remember. Like I said before, having a memory like this can be just as much a gift and a curse. The first weight loss era lasted about 5 years. I found love in three. Real honest-to-goodness love. I experienced a broken heart and a lifetime of love all in one year. It took the full year, but it ended up being the worst and best year of my life. Worst because of the real heartache Kathy caused me and best because of the wonderful life Eileen has given me. The two don't compare in any way. But I guess knowing what true heartbreak and love loss felt like made me hopeful that I could love again. It took almost a whole year, but I was lucky to find it. And you think we could have had more time if I wasn't so in love with Kathy. If I had known how it was going to turn out Kathy and I would have never gotten together. It would have caused me so little pain over the years. I loved Kathy. I do not doubt that I always would have wondered what if I hadn't gotten together with her what it would have been like to love her. Even if it wasn't obvious that she didn't love me as much as I loved her. I think deep down she did love me but wouldn't let herself admit it because the upheaval in her life would have been monumental.

The reason I tell you all about this in a book about my life losing and gaining weight is would Kathy have stayed with me or even remained faithful when I gained weight? She was big into physical fitness so maybe I would have never gained the weight back. But if I did, would she have stayed with me? I would hope she would have. But then again, she seemed to be ok with cheating on her fiancé once with me. Would I always worry about her doing the same to me? I never had that doubt about Eileen. Only in my insecurities did I imagine Eileen having an affair. First, we spent just about every minute together from the time we were married. I won't say where we spent most of our time together, but we were horizontal most of the time. Then the kids came and the time for any kind of an affair disappeared for her and me. I would gain and lose weight over the next 30-plus years, but she was always here for me. I would have always wondered if I gained weight would Kathy have wandered? She had seemed, in my eyes to love me but was so confused, maybe because she was in love with two guys at the same time and took the easy way out. Get rid of the one you haven't been together with the longest. That was me. So, I got the short end of the stick again, and she walked away probably happy that she didn't have to think about it anymore. I walked away wondering if I'd ever recover. Turns out that not only did Kathy make the right decision for me in the long run, but she also probably made the wrong one for herself. I love hard. And I loved my kids with all my heart. Now I have two grandchildren and it makes me happy that the big guy in the sky gave me enough time on this earth to have them in my life too. Unfortunately, for Kathy's family, she died way too young. I always had hoped we could have gotten together later in life just to find out why she did what she did and if it was hard for her or just a second thought. Hindsight is always 20/20 but I'd still like to know if I did something wrong to drive her away or if the guilt just got to her. When she pulled the plug, we ended on a very high note, so I'm still and always will be confused as to what I did wrong or if she just got scared about how much she felt for me during the vacation we took. If that were the case, I would think she'd have gone the other way. These are all statements that have plagued me for most of my life. Not because I feel like I should have married Kathy, but because of the unknown. If she had given me a reason why she did all that just to leave me in the end, I probably could have lived the rest of my life with less aggravation. When we did meet one time for lunch, we only had about 20 minutes and after we got through all the pleasantries, we started to talk about our kids. After all that was done, she had to go back to the emergency room, and I had to go back to the echo lab.

The next day I called her to see if she wanted to have lunch again. She immediately said yes. I said what time do you want to meet me down in the cafeteria? She said "they will let you come down to St. Bernard for lunch?" St. Bernard was about 30 blocks away and would take me the 30 minutes I was allotted for lunch just to get there. I asked my boss if I could take an hour or so for lunch to meet an old friend. He wasn't very good on his own although he did spend many a day taking more than half an hour for lunch and refused to let me go. I called Kathy back and said I couldn't make it. I asked her when she would be back at Michael Reese, and she said she was done there. I told her I really wanted to keep this lunch date because there are things, I really needed to know about us that would help my sanity. I think that scared her. She was willing to talk about the things in the present, but I think she was hesitant to talk about the past. I never got to have that lunch. Even later in our lives when we reconnected over a patient, I wanted her to see that is a friend of mine. She said she'd be happy to see him, but she had a three-month waiting list. This gave me the obvious idea that she must be one hell of a doctor to have a 3-month waiting list. She was known for her holistic approach to solving intestinal problems. She took time to listen to patients and wasn't one of those doctors that ran in, gave you a prescription, and then ran out. I never saw her as a patient, but I'm quoting comments from her website. Although the end of a relationship can be so painful it spans a generation, I don't look at it negatively anymore. I still have so many questions, but they will have to wait till I see her again.

Chapter 24

How many more years of pain are you willing to endure?

So, how long have you been on this journey? Has it been all your life like

me? Small spans of months getting so close to your goal only to tip the other way and go back to the weight you started at or gain even more? I read an article one time that stated going up and down in weight is actually more detrimental than staying at one weight. That weight may be 250 pounds for you. That's where your body wants to be. If you're over six feet and are built naturally big, 250 might be a normal weight for you. You may have the ultimate dad bod, but that's ok. If that's where you are supposed to be, try to stay there. Because as you age you almost always are less physical. Before you know it, you can start creeping up higher. 250 becomes 275 and then 300. And it can happen fast. It's the same thing for women. You may start at 120 when you are young. Just like 220 was for me. You stayed at that weight or around it for most of your life. You marry at 26 and have your first child at 28. You gain 60 pounds with the pregnancy. Which can happen and you shouldn't be upset about that. The baby wanted you to eat so you ate. Now the bouncing baby girl comes into the world. You lose weight right after the baby comes. But you're so busy with the baby. She's colicky. You're up for most of the night with your bundle of joy. You sleep when she sleeps. You drop 40 pounds but stall there. So, your normal weight is 140 now. You know it's higher than it should be, but you have a wonderful husband who loves you more than air and it doesn't matter to him. But when you look in the mirror it bothers you. The baby gets a little older and now you're chasing a toddler. Your husband works a lot. You have a regular schedule and drop the baby off at daycare and have to pick her up after work because your husband may not be home till 7:00 PM. He helps with the baby when he gets home. You want to spend time with him too. You all go to bed at 9:00 because you're both exhausted. You fall asleep in .04 seconds. You get up the next day and start the whole routine over again. The extra 20 pounds you have retained stays. You eat like a normal person, but you don't really pay close attention to what you eat. You and your husband have a lot of takeouts because it's just easier. After the baby turns 3 you notice that you have crept up to 150. Then surprise! You're pregnant! This time you gain less weight during the pregnancy. Let's say 40 pounds. You immediately lose 20 pounds but now you're dropping off two kids, teaching 25 kids all day, and rushing to the daycare center to pick up your kids because your husband is now working till 8:00 pm. Because he's moved up the corporate ladder and works hard to make a lot of money for the family. He is missing out because he has no idea that making money isn't as important as being with your children. You have a bigger house and a nicer SUV for bringing the kids to daycare. But you still don't have time to do anything but teach and watch kids. Sometimes your husband doesn't make it home until the kids are in bed. You find yourself snacking a little more than before. Now you're at 165 and you hate the way you look and feel. Your husband is absolutely no help at all. He even works most Saturdays now too. You move to an even bigger house. Your husband is a VP of Operations of the company. Now it's not unusual for him to go in on Sunday too. He may only be there for 4 hours, but it's not helping. He flops down on Sunday at 12:30 and starts watching football. He's not paying attention to the kids, or you and you have now got a 7-day-a-week job raising children. You want to start going to a gym and exercising but there is no time to go. Your husband still loves you but doesn't make love to you as much as he used to. You fight more than you usually do. He starts to question what you do all day and why can't you work out. This completely fries you and you are so mad at him that the coldness is evident almost every day. You finally sit down with him and say do you want to get back down to normal weight and if you need more help from him. He decides the best way to do this is to buy you a $2000.00 treadmill for the basement that you can get on when the babies sleep. No problem, right? Wrong. You work full-time even though you don't have to. You love your job. You love your class. It's fun for you. You have to get a babysitter on conference night because you know your husband won't be home in time to watch the kids. The new treadmill has dust on it because you just don't have the time. You make a new commitment to exercise. The only time you have is at night. So, when your husband gets home you practically toss the kids at him and go downstairs. You don't care how tired he is. He must find a way to be a better father and husband. Part of this weight problem is his fault too. He hasn't given you the support to help you lose weight. Now it's your turn. You have to fight for your health. He's not happy having to do something other than have dinner and go to bed but you need your time. You change the way you eat. You work hard to get back down to 140. That's fantastic. But you are still not happy. You want to be at 120 again. But your body won't allow you to get that low. Your body has changed because of the kids. You make it down to 135. You are excited! And you should be! You've done a great job. You are ok with the small amount of extra weight. Then guess what happens? You pee on the stick and the plus side appears. Surprise! Now your depressed because you know the weight will creep up some during the pregnancy. Now you have knowledge about how to eat and how to stay away from snacks and you don't gain as much this time but you are at 150 when you deliver. You're back down to 140 after a month. Now with three kids, you have no time for anything. You creep back up to 150 then 160. You are unhappy and it's affecting every aspect of your life. You are trying to eat healthily. The weight now hovers around 145. You are still not happy but it will have to do.

Chapter 26

Why did it happen?

What I described above is something that men will never understand. Having children changes a woman's body. Women can sometimes get back down to their original weight but only if they have a good support system in place. He could have made VP a couple of years later and you could have stayed in the 2500 sq. foot house instead of the 4000 sq. foot house. Just one or two extra hours a night would have been all she needed. Now he has a very unhappy wife, and his life isn't good either. What went wrong here? It's not a big, confusing answer. Lack of communication. Ambition. Carving out time for yourself. Having a perceptive partner. This is some of the examples.

There are more. Let's look at a man's path. And mind you this is just one of many paths.

Scott is thin from the time he is 18 after being obese for many years. He makes a commitment to himself that he was no longer going to put up with the pain of being rejected by the opposite sex. Scott is also tired of being out of shape. Scott's weight doesn't stop him, but it doesn't help him either. Scott talks to a friend one night after drinking at a party. Bill offers to help Scott get in shape. He commits to showing up at the gym every morning at 6:00 am to help Scott get in shape. Scott commits and promises Bill that he will be there every day except Sunday for as long as it takes. Scott spends time reading a book called "The Atkins Diet" and takes everything in. The book talks about rapid weight loss if you stick to the diet. Scott is there on the first day with Bill waiting outside in the parking lot at the gym. As they go in, Bill says "this is going to take some time. You can do this. Just promise me you'll stick with it." Scott does and also knows that you don't break a promise to Bill. For 6 months Scott sticks with the low-carb high protein diet and weight lifts with Bill for an hour and a half each day. He showers and goes right to work. Scott stays with the diet and the weight drops off quickly. The first 20 pounds come off in 3 weeks. It goes on this way until Scott reaches 210 pounds from an original 290 pounds. He drops an extra 10 pounds but finds he feels better at 210. He feels strong and confident. He is still hesitant around women after years of rejection. He reminds himself too often about those rejections and it holds him back in the beginning. But he gets the nerve up to ask a really pretty girl he works with to go out with him. Kim says yes and that starts the ball rolling. The relationship doesn't last long, but the confidence Scott feels doubles. He quickly finds a girl that is as willing to be with him as he is with her. Surprisingly, she's the ex-girlfriend of the guy Kim left me for. Call it Karma, but it was wonderful to be with her. She is in a rebound phase and because Scott doesn't understand what that means, he just goes along with it. But Scott is not deterred.

He has more confidence than ever and the more nurses he interacts with, the more go out with him. Scott even gets the girl he wanted in high school. Unfortunately, she's a rebound too. You would think Scott would have learned from the first time. Apparently not. For 2 years this goes on until Scott falls in love with a dangerous woman. One that has the potential to shatter him. But Scott can resist this long-haired brunette with the most beautiful blue eyes. She is Scott's dream girl. Loaded with personality, and athletic talent and Scott and Kathy are great as friends. Scott wants more, the problem is simple. Kathy is engaged to another man. Kathy and Scott continue to play racquetball and golf together all the time. After many months of this, they have a fun evening on a Friday night when her fiancé is out of town. Kathy goes with him to have an evening of racquetball, Dinner, and a trip to a bar for dancing. When Kathy and Scott leave the bar Scott leans in to kiss Kathy on the cheek to say thank you for the fun night. At the last minute, Kathy turns her head and Scott kisses her on the lips. He says he is sorry saying "I was aiming for your cheek." Kathy grabs Scott around the neck and pulls him in for a long, deep, passionate kiss. Scott almost wets his pants he's so excited. When they finish the kiss they rest their foreheads together, allowing Scott to say "Do you know how long I've waited for that to happen?" Kathy says, "Shut up and recline the seats." I do that immediately and 2 hours later, we finally finish and decide it's time to go home. Kathy still lives at home, and so does Scott so they have limited areas to make love. They seem to manage just fine, though. Motel rooms, times when their parents are away, and weekends away when she doesn't need to be with her fiancé. Scott and Kathy live in an era before cell phones so they can disappear into the day or night, and no one can find us.

Chapter 27

Things are complicated

Scott wants to marry Kathy. But she's not interested in breaking up with her fiancé. She just wants two men at the same time. Scott is getting very frustrated but takes out all his anger in the gym to help maintain muscle mass. Kathy and Scott go on vacation together to Las Vegas and then drive to California from there. They spend a lot of time in bed and Scott feels like he's finally making her see that she would be better with him. On the second to the last day of their vacation, Kathy feels so guilty she flies home early without Scott saying "I can't do this anymore." Scott is heartbroken. But he's also very angry. Scott doesn't want to be in the same room with Kathy and being that they work together, this is a problem. Everyone in the department knows what's going on. Scott and Kathy think they have kept their love affair secret, but it's obvious to both of them that it's not. 3 weeks later after Scott starts dating every woman he can because he's so angry, Kathy asks to meet him after work. Scott says ok and at 5:00 they meet at an ice cream place. Kathy tells Scott that he's dating all these women and she is getting very jealous. Scott loses it and starts to yell at Kathy saying "I only want you. If you break off your engagement, I'll buy you a new ring the very next day. Scott tells Kathy how much he loves her. She says "You're just infatuated with me." Scott says "Don't tell me what love is. I'm a big boy and I know that I'm in love with you. They walk away with nothing settled except the fact that Scott knows he's getting to her with all the other girls. All of them really mean nothing to Scott. But the day finally comes, and Kathy marries the wrong guy. Scott doesn't go to the wedding or reception because he doesn't think he can hold his tongue.

All this time Scott has maintained the weight and even lost some of it because of his loss of appetite because he's so upset. He takes his anger out on the weights at the gym. For about 6 months Scott continues to bring women down to the department just to piss off Kathy. Even after she's married, she can't stay in the same room when Scott has a girlfriend in there with him. It's just painful for everyone to watch. Kathy finally can't take it anymore and puts in her two-week notice. On her last day, a party is planned to send her off. Scott calls in sick and rides his motorcycle from southwest of Chicago all the way to Iowa for no reason other than to be as far away from that party as possible. He goes over the Mississippi and then turns around, gets gas, and drives all the way back. He missed everything. She didn't even leave him a note.

The fight continues on the weight front as Scott has his first bout of mild depression after the breakup. He loses interest in the gym and starts to drink a lot of beer. When he gets on the scale and notices that he has gained 25 pounds back he immediately changes his ways and goes back to his normal routine. The depression fades and he feels confident again. Many women after Kathy have been with Scott. It's been 10 months since she left when the girl he was dating just before Kathy loses her mother to a rare lung disease. Scott has thought a lot about her because the month they had together was hot and heavy and they just clicked. But Scott ruined it by falling for an engaged woman he loved. Scott's mother talked him into going to Eileen's mother's funeral wear he apologized about how things ended. He said he wanted to go out and explain everything to her so maybe they can start over. Scott knows he's caught her at a weak moment, but that's something that his Kids will razz him about in the future until he dies. When Eileen hears the whole story, she's glad that it happened because she'll never have to worry about her again. Scott likes her attitude and falls in love with her so quickly they end up getting married in 5 months after Scott gives Eileen the engagement ring, they are married. Just for fun Scott invites Kathy to the wedding and she actually shows up with her husband. I sing a beautiful romantic song to Eileen on stage. Scott looks up just in time to see Kathy practically running out of the room. She doesn't get back until way after the song is over. She has red-rimmed eyes but I think I'm the only one who notices. At the end of the wedding, Kathy corners Scott as everyone's leaving. She looks at him and says, "We have to leave." she is looking down and seems upset. I pull her chin up and say "this was your choice, Kathy. This could have all been for you. Now I love Eileen more than anything or anyone."

Kathy nods and starts to say something. It sounds like I made a mistake, but she walks away when she says it. Scott just shakes his head and goes find the love of his life. The one that lasts 38 years as of the writing of this book. She is still everything to Scott.

Chapter 28

Life goes on

Why do I go into this whole story is because, as John Mellencamp said "Oh yeah, life goes on. Long after the thrill of living is gone." I had all those years as a thin, young man. I thought everything would be perfect when I lost weight. Bad and good things happen. And life goes on. Marriage has been good to me, but not to my weight. Like I said before things happen that will challenge you. Those challenges may affect your weight.

I went back to school after I got married. 8 hours a day 5 days a week. With an added 3 to 4 hours of homework a night. Why does this matter? This is a receipt for gaining weight. Sitting around, snacking on anything I could get my hands on. Back to drinking almost a gallon of milk a day. Smoking 2 packs of cigarettes a day. I gained 50 pounds during school. Then we wanted to have a baby and I didn't want to have the baby around cigarette smoke. So, I quit smoking. 2 packs a day down to nothing. It was brutal. But I knew it needed to be done. So, three years after we got married, I gained all the weight back. Back to 290. How fair was that to Eileen? She really must have and still does love me because it's been a rollercoaster of weight gain and loss. I have been all the way back to 230 and as high as 384. Yes, I said 384. I lost 80 pounds at that time so I could have a knee replacement without the problem of supporting myself. But after the knee problems finally wear taken care of, I went right back up to 390. My body started to fail and I knew I had to do something drastic.

I went to a bariatric surgeon because I needed just a little more hope. The depression was bad. I was embarrassed to be seen outside. Swimming was out of the question. I was worried that my kids wear embarrassed about having me as a father. And Eileen. How fair was it to her? She has to look at me naked. Something I am totally embarrassed about. She says she still loves me no matter what I look like. She's just extremely worried about my health. Big time worried. I'm short of breath with any significant exertion. It was time to do something drastic before I hit 400 pounds.

I had a gastric sleeve procedure on the 29 of June of that year. Was it easy, no. It was a painful surgery? at times. Anytime they cut more than half of your stomach out, things will hurt. But talk about cutting your appetite in half or more. And back to the high protein, low carb diet again. I drink a lot of protein shakes. Chicken breasts become my closes friend turned enemy. I still like them, but sometimes they get old. I found the list I was looking for about weight loss after the surgery. January 29 was the surgery. I weighed 380 pounds. On 7/9 I was down 31 pounds. I was on a protein shake regimen during that time. 7/16 338, 7/19 335, 7/30 328, 8/12 324, 8/26 314, 8/31 314, 9/24 304, 10/14 291, 10/30 280 and it goes down from there to my current weight which is about 265. I hit what they call a wall. I wasn't drinking the shakes anymore. So little to no protein. I found these granola bars that I really liked and would use as a snack when I was hungry. That kind of got out of hand. My goal was 250. As of the writing of this book, I am starting over with the higher protein low carb diet again to hit that goal. It will take a little time, but with a change in habit I will do it. My stomach is still very small, so my meal portions are still small too. I fell off the wagon as so many people do. Something as small as granola bars covered in peanut butter can be a determinant to my weight loss goals. It is a little thing. A 160-calorie granola bar that when you snack on all day, can add up to an easy 1200 calorie mistake. Right now, I'm writing this at 3:00 am. I've eaten 4 of those granola bars already. I sometimes have trouble sleeping. I usually do a lot of writing at this time. But it can be a dangerous time for me to be awake because I eat the equivalent of a full meal just because I'm awake and bored. I need to sleep till morning. If I could sleep until 6:30 am I'll have a much better day. So even though I write a significant amount at this time of night, I'd rather be sleeping.

Chapter 29

Remember those assholes who made fun of you?

Let's hope you run into one of them after you lose all the weight. There is nothing more satisfying than running into one of these people. Maybe someone from high school (those are the best ones because that's when the cruelty is the most hateful). Those are the best ones. Sometimes you'll see them look at you and they know you but because they were such an asshole to you in high school, they don't want to even approach you because you've changed so much. I guess you must have the mean gene to make that work. The mean gene is a chromosome that seems to appear in a lot of these people. The real nasty need to make fun of the lesser people in the world. The short, the tall, the fat, the people with acne, the special needs kids, and the autistic kids that these people seem to have no problem making fun of. I'm not only talking about high schoolers. The high schoolers turn into college students doing the same thing. And then they turn into mean adults, who like to belittle people who work under them. The cashier in the grocery store who is nasty to everyone because she dropped out of college and is now stuck at the register at the grocery store. And when guys like me, the ones she made fun of when she was a cheerleader, come through the line and pay for the groceries with an American Express Black Card. It hasn't happened to me. I don't make enough money to have a black card. But it's happened to someone out there. And every overweight person that was made fun of should have been there to witness it. It's the same thing with people who have terrible acned when they are a teenager. They hit their early twenties and the acne goes away. Suddenly, you've got a good-looking guy or girl that was terrorized in high school for their "Pizza face" starring in a Hollywood blockbuster and you were the one who made fun of that person in high school. You're now running a non-profit and could sure use their help with a donation. As soon as they see your name on the letterhead the letter gets filed under "No f-ing way." People like us remember the hurt you caused us. You may not think it was traumatic for us or you may be under the influence of the "I was just kidding" thought process. By the way, no one is just kidding. Behind that statement is always a little bit of how the person feels about you. They may not be conscious of it, but it's there.

Chapter 30

Fat shaming is a relatively new term used to describe those people who feel like it's within their right to not only make fun of people but also make suggestions to someone overweight like "why don't you just eat less and exercise more?" or "It's so simple. Stop eating junk and go jogging!" or a personal favorite "We're so concerned about you, you're going to die early." Now, this last one I can completely discard because I have treated more overweight old people than you'd ever believe. I have also watched a marathon runner in the Chicago marathon years ago die in front of me because of over exertion during a very hot day. She was in her forties and in good shape. It wasn't her first marathon. I've also seen professional sports players with heart disease bad enough to force retirement. No one really knows who is going to present as unhealthy.

Before I had my knees replaced I could run on a treadmill during a stress test for twelve minutes. Here is the bruce protochol for a stress test done for patients at hospitals. It list's grade and speed of the treadmill at 3 minute intervals. Here is a chart explaining the different stages of a Bruce protocol stress test.

Bruce Treadmill Test Stages, Speeds, and Inclines

Stage	Treadmill Speed	Treadmill Incline
1	1.7 mph	10% grade
2	2.5 mph	12% grade
3	3.4 mph	14% grade
4	4.2 mph	16% grade
5	5.0 mph	18% grade
6	5.5 mph	20% grade
7	6.0 mph	22% grade

So I, as a fat guy, was able to reach the end of stage 4. I was over 300 pounds at the time. I had no ekg changes and the test was considered normal. When I was getting ready for the test my co worker in the echo lab said I wouldn't go past stage 2 because I was so fat. Another example of fat shaming. As you can see, I was able to complete stage 4 at 4.2 mph at a 16% grade. Most treadmills in health clubs do not go past a 10% grade. Fat people can be in pretty good shape. Look at football players on the offensive line. These are the big guys in front of the quarterback who protect him from being sacked. (crushed). the two heaviest current NFL linemen are **Daniel Faalele** (6-feet-9, 380 pounds) of the Baltimore Ravens and Trent Brown (6-8, 380) of the New England Patriots. These are elite athletes who are performing at an unbelievable level of speed and strength. Yes, they are very tall too. But there are offensive linemen that are 6'3" and 340 pounds and can still stop a much faster linebacker from sacking a quarterback. Not every heavy person is out of shape. These guys still get fat shamed probably on a weekly basis. Some reporter will ask "don't you think you'd be faster if you lost 40 pounds?" Like this skinny little reporter knows that it will help the player be better. If a 6'8" 380-pound guy from the NFL came at me because I had the nerve to call him a fat pig he could catch me in less than 20 seconds and pummel me into dust. And I'm 275 pounds.

One other thing we should cover in fat shaming is someone who is overweight calling someone who is heavier than them names or offering advice on how to lose weight. This person does not need your advice. If you have lost a lot of weight and the person is interested in how you did it then it's ok to give them the information in a nice, informative way. I would even pull them to the side to tell them that I had the Gastric Sleeve surgery. I would take the time to explain the procedure and the risks and the way you have to eat after the surgery. All that information should be given in a professional, kind way. You are conveying a bit of information. Not offering an opinion unless you're asked for it.

Try really hard not to fat-shame anyone. It's none of your business to know why a person is overweight. Nor is it your privilege to express your opinion on how they can lose weight.

Chapter 31

To continue on fat shaming there is one other type of fat shaming that goes on regularly. It is prejudice plain and simple. Somewhere, years ago, someone got it in their head that if you are overweight you must be lazy. You discriminate when you come to this conclusion. I'm sure I was passed over for promotions and jobs because I was overweight even though I was more qualified than any other candidate. I consistently did more echocardiographic studies than most other techs I was working with. I'm not bragging. It was a simple fact. I just saw a cardiologist that I worked with many years ago. My wife Eileen was in the room with me when he said, "you were the hardest working echo tech I've every had the pleasure of working with." He has been a cardiologist for over 35 years. That was one of the best compliments I ever received. I was also overweight at that time. I would really like to thank Dr. S for such a fantastic compliment.

The amazing thing to me regarding this type of predigest, Is that people, news organizations, weight loss companies, and many other health-related magazines assume that every single person on this earth is not happy with their body because they are fat. There are paraplegics that were extremely anger with their body image right after their accident or illness that now may be happy with their body image. It probably took time, but it does happen. These people still have to defend themselves all the time because certain places discriminate against handicapped people. A significant number of government buildings in this country do not have handicapped ramps or elevators. This is pure discrimination and makes the person in the wheelchair feel either angry or depressed because no one in their state government thinks that giving access to all people in the state access to public records or even library books.

    By no means am I comparing the severity of a paraplegic's journey as compared to an overweight person. Paraplegics are forced in usually one day to go from a normal walking person to being confined to a wheelchair. But yet, an overweight person may suffer the same level of depression as a person in a wheelchair. There is an extremely high amount of depression in overweight people. Especially in those who are consistently fat-shamed. I mentioned before that I had made some psychologists wealthy just by the amount of time I spent on their couches. Many overweight teenagers attempt suicide because of constant bullying. Now that the American Medical Association has classified obesity as a disease, a number of people should accept their friend or co-worker as having a disease instead of being lazy. My psychologist has tried to get me to understand that the majority of people in this country don't classify obesity as a disease. So, their archaic view on obesity or overweight people has to change before fat-shaming becomes a non-factor. I have always thought that people would just treat all overweight people with the dignity that they treat their trim friends. To look at the person you know at work or with friends and respect them as a normal person. A person that makes you laugh, or is always kind to you, or goes out of their way to make sure you are treated well. It's doesn't always mean they have the hots for you, it means that they are a good person. People who are overweight are pleasers. They try to make up for their looks by being nice to everyone. Obviously, this isn't always true. There are jerks that are overweight. I had bosses that were significantly overweight who were total assholes. Pardon the bad word but nothing else describes them. Some people are just mean. They are usually people who were once skinny and gained weight later in life. They assume it's ok to continue their bad behavior so being overweight doesn't matter to them. If it's a guy we're talking about they will still feel like they have the looks that get the ladies to want to be with them. If you are a victim of one of these idiots stand your ground. Don't let a jerk make you do something you don't want to do just because he's the boss. Go over his head and file a complaint. Power-hungry people push the boundaries quite often. Ask that your complaint remain anonymous. These kinds of people are just bullies with power. If this person is the owner of the company, then it's time to get a new job.

Sorry, off on another tangent. I have to go with what strikes me at the moment. Usually, it's a memory of someone I knew. So, it's relevant to this weight journey book.

Chapter 31

This section is for older teens and adults. If you are younger than this I ask that you please wait to read this until you're at least 16. You'll understand what this chapter means when you're older. So please move on to the next chapter so you can get the full value of this book. Please do this for me.

Most of the time, a person who is heavy will make a great friend or even a lover. I know when I was heavy long before I lost the weight, I knew more about the female anatomy than any of my guy friends. I knew what to do if I got a woman to make love to me. If this would have happened in high school, the girl would have been completely satisfied because I knew what I was doing and how to make a woman remember making love to me. Knowing about how to have sex and please your partner is so important. You will be better than any other partner that person has ever had. They will stay with you just because of you. Your willingness to please your partner first. I just wanted one serious girlfriend that I would be with long enough for us to lose our virginity. I had gone to the library to examine the female anatomy so I knew where and what to touch and what else I could use to bring a woman pleasure. I just needed the girl and I would have been fine and so would she. So I'd like to send an angry note to all the girls from the junior and senior classes for not recognizing me as a possible sex God:

Dear girls,

How you all missed out. How you missed orgasm after orgasm if you had just taken a chance and dated a fat guy. A fat guy who was so enamored with sex that the first girl I lost my virginity to had 3 orgasms before I got mine. Three with a capital T. I was relentless. This could have been you! I think I'm going to have to name names. You should know who you are. Because if you had just said yes, we would have had such fun. So let's go with a list. I'm sure I'll forget some of you, but if you ever caught me following you in the hallway, looking down at your butt, consider yourself on the list. The list goes from the most wanted one to the most wanted one. No, that's not a typo. Any one of you could have been my favorite.

1. Barb T.
2. Tammi T.
3. Melissa E.
4. Cheryl W.
5. Kathy E.
6. Erica W.
7. Laura H.
8. Mary S.
9. Shirley B.
10. Jill C.
11. Sue B.
12. Leslie G.
13. Kim W.
14. Dawn E.
15. Betty L.

So there you go. The girls that missed out. God if you only knew how ready I was for one of you to get just drunk enough at a party to say "you know, that Scott seems like he would know what he's doing." If I had it back I would have walked around the school with a shirt on that said "I can find the clitoris." Maybe 5 shirts. One for each day. Maybe that one thing would have been enough to get some attention. But instead, I wore regular clothes, carried a bunch of extra weight, and let people make fun of me. That's probably the reason you all stayed away. Someone called me fat Moss in front of you so I was automatically a no-go. What a shame for all of you. All I would have needed was an hour. Really, just an hour.

This section is for Barb T. You were the one. The one that I would have pulled all the stops out. I just wish the time we did have together wasn't scared by Rick and Terri. You knew that I would do anything for you and often did. Maybe I should have been more persuasive. I never wanted to push you. I wanted you to pick me. I don't know what stopped you from making a move. It's obvious to me now that I should have just gone for it. I made a huge mistake and it cost me. It cost me the opportunity to show you how much you meant to me. I was so worried about making you mad that I missed my opportunity to make you crazy. I hope you know now how I felt about you.

Love,
Scott

Awwww! Wasn't that sweet? I hope none of you threw up during that rant. But I do have a point. I might have had a chance with any of these girls. But I decided I liked Little Debbie better than all of them. She had a lot to offer. I told you all the treats she had. None of the girls on the list gave me a starcrunch treat. Little Debbie handed out treats like crazy. I should have divorced her in my sophomore year. Then I would have been thin for my junior and senior years. I could have found one girl on my list that would have gone out with me.

Chapter 32

For my young readers

So lets get back to strict weight loss. What do you see in your future? Because now is the time for you to act. If you're in 7th grade and you have been made fun of since you were in grade school for being heavy than it's time to act. What are you, 13? Here's what were going to do. First things first. Talk to you mom and dad. Or if you only have one parent talk to her or him. You need there help! They will do the grocery shopping and if you can, ask them if you can pick out the foods to help you lose weight. Then we're going to do this:

1. Stay out of the cereal and bread aisle.
2. The family may need bread but you don't.
3. You need meat. Bacon is ok, bolonia is ok. (put one slice of bolonia on a paper plate, but a piece of sandwich cheese on top of that, then put another piece of bolonia on top of that. Bolonia and cheese sandwich without the bread. (Bring a napkin)
4. Vegetables. Find some you like. They make mixed vegetables if you would prefer that to eating raw vegetables. But I have to tell you, raw carrots are an easy snack. You don't even have to peel them. Just make sure you wash them off good.
5. Ask your mom or dad to make things like hamburgers and cheeseburgers for you without the bun. Meatloaf with spices and at least one egg mixed up together is also good. Were going to cheat a little here just to make the meatloaf a little better... half a cup of dried bread crumbs. Spread throughout an entire meatloaf it isn't that bad. It will help hold the meatloaf together along with the egg. Don't forget to get a bottle of steak seasoning and use about a tablespoon of it for a two pound meat loaf. You can season it to taste. If one tablespoon isn't enough try two the next time.
6. Fruit. Some fruit is high in sugar. Strawberries are higher than let say watermelon although I'm not positive on that. But for a treat when you come home from school, slice up 4 strawberries after you clean them and put a tablespoon of cool whip on top. You'll love the taste and it won't stop your weight loss.
7. Buy some good, flavorful cheese. I love extra sharp cheddar. Pick whatever you like but try to stay away from the processed stuff. Get real cheese. It will also get you through

the day. Snack on a couple of pieces of cheese when you're hungry

8. Remember. You are going to be hungry most of the time. Tough it out! Being hungry is part of losing weight. You have to drink a lot of water so you feel full most of the day. Remember, the bathroom is your friend. Be close to one so you can run in to pee every 30 minutes or so. If you tell your teachers privately about what you're doing, they will excuse you to go to the bathroom during class. If they won't call me. I come an kick their butt. If they really won't, go anyway and then explain your diet to the principle. The principle will talk to the teacher.

9. Remember the main food groups for this weight loss program. High protein low carbohydrates and low sugar. That basically means meat, eggs, cheese, vegetables, some lite fruit, and lots of water. You can also have protein shakes. They will take away the hunger and replace a whole meal. Try to get the pre mixed, individual shakes. These aren't that cheap. But they do replace a whole meal so explain that to your parents. Replacing an entire meal with a two dollar shake may be cheaper for them than all the other stuff you would have eaten in a regular meal. My lunch is always a protein shake now. It's incredibly easy and is loaded with good stuff. Just about any flavor you can think of. I like plain vanilla. But I have had chocolate, chocolate peanut butter, Cookies and cream, just about anything you can think of. You can get cases of protein drinks at some of the large warehouse stores too.

10. This is going to take some time. You have to be willing to stick with this. You also have to be willing to lift some weights. And also take a walk. Find a track at the local high school or just go to the mall and walk around if it's winter.

Start with 20 minutes at a good pace. Work your way up to an hour if you can. It will be great for your heart and will also, just by moving more, help burn calories. Facebook marketplace or offer up are both good places to find older used weights to buy for a cheap price. You can get something close to you so you and your parents can go pick them up. Start off with low weight and a lot of reps. Than slowly move the weight up but keep up with the reps. The more reps you do, the more defined your muscles with be. Don't forget sit-ups and push ups. Try to do as many as you can. If that's only 2 that's ok. Withing a week you'll be up to 3. Soon, you'll be pumping them out as fast as you can. You only have to work out for a half an hour to an hour to help with the weight loss.

All of these steps should be cleared with your doctor. But I know a lot of you won't. Please try to clear it if you can. Mainly the exercise stuff. Most docs believe in a low calorie approach to weight loss. That can work too, but it takes longer. Don't overdue it with the exercise. Take things slow. If you are an adult watch for signs of a heart attack. If you start having chest pain that goes into the left arm STOP EXERCISING! Sit down and if the pain doesn't go away call an ambulance. This is not something to mess with! Being thin is wonderful. Being dead, not so much.

Chapter 33

Let's finish this up

You now have options. Several of them. This is going to suck. There is no other way to put it. You will have to work very hard to get to your goal. Staying at that goal can sometimes be harder. But remember, there are major rewards on the other side of fat. (I still hate that word) If you're a girl. Think about how nice it would be to be a size 6 or 8? To pick out any fashion you want and be able to find it in your size. And then there are the boys. They will be pretty boys, and they will want to go out with you! No more third wheel. Just you and him. Think about gym class. Being able to keep up with all the other girls during class. They want you to play soccer, you can do it. Softball? Sure. How about dodgeball? Why not. Find one of the girls that used to make fun of you and pummel them with the ball. It will be so much fun! But remember to stick with the friends you had when you were overweight. Those are your true friends. Not the click of girls that invites you in there inner circle. You know, the gossip hounds. Stay as far away from those girls as you can. Trust me. It's just better this way.

    Now you guys. The weight you lose will come off fast if you stick to this program if you want to call it that. Four words. High protein, low carbohydrates. If you stick with that and throw in some weight lifting, you will be amazed at the amount of weight you'll lose. Stick with it until you need a new belt, and pants, and shirts. All of that stuff. If your feet shrink that's a whole other problem. Go see an orthopedic surgeon. Now lets think of the girls. Let's say your a sophomore in high school and school has just ended. You now have about three months to lose a lot of weight. Set yourself up with some weights in the basement or even outside. If you life in an apartment don't drop the weights! You'll get a visit from the landlord and that's never fun. Walk outside even if it's hot as hell. Take a water bottle with you so you remain hydrated. Try to work your way up to a mile a day. Take Sundays off but the rest of the days are on you. You want to lose weight so some girl you've been falling all over for the last two years will actually notice you. When you're ready, ask her out. If it only took you the three months to lose all the weight, she just might say yes. But you'll never know until you ask her. Have the guts to do so. If she turns you down when your thin, it wasn't meant to be. So move on to the next contestant on the weight is right! Some girl is going to be so impressed with the way you look and because you were once overweight, you will probably be a funny guy that makes all the girls and guys laugh. That's because you needed that sense of humor to fit in with all the skinny kids. Now your thin and you still have that fantastic sense of humor. Some girl will love the idea of going out with you. They know that you will be fun to be with and now you look just like Justin Timberlake. Ok maybe that's a stretch. You'll be more confident, be willing to stand up for yourself, and your own self astem will be through the roof. Just don't let it go to your head. Remember too that the kids that were your friends before you lost the weight are still your friends. Not the knucklehead jocks or pretty boys. Guys can have clicks too. Try to stay away from those. Have fun now that you are at a good weight. If you still have more to go, remember that your day is coming if you just stick with it.

Now I want to talk to the Morbidly Obese men and women that are out there. Like me, I feel your pain. I was there. Probably still fit in the obese category. But I'm so much healthier than I was. My final solution was the bariatric sleeve surgery that I had. It's a last stop on your weight loss journey. If you are Morbidly Obese you need to look into this as an option. I'm talking about those people who are way up there. Maybe 75 to 150 pounds overweight. Even more in some cases. This surgery forces you to eat less. You will experience pain if you overeat. It sucks. My protions have become very small compared to what they use to be. I am an italian food lover. Pasta is high in carbs. But a little pasta with meatsause makes me happy and I have a tendency to dance around for my wife when she makes it. And who can resist a 275 pound guy dancing around in ballet shoes. She's all over me after that. There was a song in the 70s that fits that thought. It is called dream weaver. That's what she would say to me if I suggested she couldn't resist me. All kidding aside, this is going to be work. Remember, for some reason the weight comes off of men faster than women. Another unequal opportunity. Just kick this things ass will you. It's time to walk into a bar and have your pick of women. Or at least have one look at you like you might be for her. It's wonderful to experience, let me tell you. Losing the weight when I was young opened so many closed doors for me (that sounded dirty). When girls came up to me after I lost all that weight and seemed to be interested in me I was extremely gun shy for a while. You need to bring your confidence up first. Allow yourself to think girls will approach you now. Or that you can approach them. It takes a little time to get there. But once your confidence is up, the flood gates open and you see what you've been missing for the last number of years. After I lost the 100 pounds post surgery I went to a bar with my wife and some friends. I dance like a old white boy. I think I was about 58 or 59. I had a 40 something girl come over to my table and ask me to dance. I gently turned her down telling her I was married and my wife was out on the dance floor. She actually said "we can dance on the other end of the dance floor so she doesn't see us." Don't worry, I still said no, but it sure was nice to be propositioned like that. I told Eileen on the way home and she bailed out of the car at 35 miles and hour and went back to kick her ass. (Big Lie). Just to be asked by someone to dance was wonderful. Eileen was actually happy for me. She new that it made me feel good to think that some much younger girl wanted to dance with me. Then she slapped me in the back of the head. I guess I was a little too happy. Just kidding. She was really happy for me.

So you've heard my story. Hopefully it won't end soon because I'd like to stick around to walk one more daughter down the aisle, watch my two boys become fathers, and my little Dana become a mother. Then I can kick the bucket and go up to heaven and find out why God made me a fat guy for most of my life. Maybe I was one of those skinny guys who use to make fun of fat kids when I was on the earth before. Payback is a bitch. I really wonder if that's how things go. You have to come down and become the person you use to make fun of when you were on earth in a previous life.

Ok. my absolute final words. You can do this. I know it sounds cliche', but you can. You just have to commit. And commit long term. Please don't subject yourself to the pain I've gone through being overweight. People are mean. We as a species have not learned how to be nice to each other. That's why we have wars, and war crimes, and skinny people who like to make fun of fat people. No we're not lazy. Yes we can be great spouses and lovers, yes we can be wealthy, and yes we can kick your ass for calling us fat. (for body slam lessons, refer to any wrestling channel).

I know how hard this will be. But you will learn to love yourself again. To be healthy, happy, and a chick or guy magnet.

As they say at Nike, Just do it! Even if you have to have surgery to make it happen. Don't forget, surgery should be your last stop on the road. You'll be glad you lost the weight. I promise.

Love
Scott Moss 2023
Copyright Scott Moss

Don't miss out!

Visit the website below and you can sign up to receive emails whenever Scott Moss publishes a new book. There's no charge and no obligation.

https://books2read.com/r/B-A-LLFTC-AQDHF

BOOKS 2 READ

Connecting independent readers to independent writers.

About the Author

Scott W. Moss was born and raised in Oak Forest, Illinois. After graduating, Scott went into the medical field, spending the next four decades helping improve lives. His ingrained sense of care and compassion translates into all he does, making him exceptional in many ways.

Scott is the consummate family man. He has been married to the love of his life for almost as long as he has worked in medicine. Together, they raised four children and now enjoy time with their grandchildren.

Milton Keynes UK
Ingram Content Group UK Ltd.
UKHW041938241124
451423UK00001BA/184